A short history of the out

and the Rheumatic Diseases

T0260586

University of California Press
Berkeley and Los Angeles, California

Cambridge University Press
London, England

© 1964 by The Regents of the University of California
Library of Congress Catalog Card Number: 64-16012

A short history of the Gout

and the Rheumatic Diseases

by W. S. C. Copeman, M.D., F.R.C.P.

There is a dead medical literature, and there is a live literature—
The dead is not all ancient, and the live is not all modern—

Oliver Wendell Holmes

UNIVERSITY OF CALIFORNIA PRESS
Berkeley and Los Angeles
1964

Foreword

Gout has long been a source of amusement to the unafflicted and a subject frequently portrayed by artists of comic and satiric bent, especially in the eighteenth and nineteenth centuries. The postures of the victims, the immense, swaddling bandages—actually shock absorbers—were bizarre if not ludicrous in appearance, and such physical attitudes of the gouty, their grimaces and cries of pain, the firm belief that such sufferers derived from the wealthy and privileged classes who had brought this fate upon themselves, appealed to the masses. The gout certainly was and remains no matter of comedy to its victims, and when it attacked those in positions of command, anguished incapacity was frequently reflected in delayed decision and activity that might ultimately affect large masses of people or even entire nations.

There are a number of reasons for studying the history of this disease. Its lineage is long if not always honorable. Effective treatment, discovered in the classical world, was lost to later ages and only recovered in comparatively recent times; the story of the search for a palliative or cure reflects the successive philosophies of medicine from credulity to science and includes almost every notable name in the history of medicine. For many centuries the illustrious victims of the disease, despite wealth and power, were condemned to the same valueless therapy employed for the gouty of lesser station, but since the great majority of cases seems to have been among the more privileged classes—at least they were more publicized—the social and political history of gout, which spans much of the

Christian Era, has been fairly well documented and provides a notable example of the influence of disease upon history.

The present work, the first full historical account of this dire ailment, was written by a distinguished rheumatologist whose scientific knowledge of gout is second to none and who, moreover, has long displayed a keen and active interest in the general history of medicine and, as will be obvious to the reader, has maintained a special concern with the history of gout and its allied ailments. He has grappled with the gout historically, scientifically, therapeutically on behalf of his patients and, it may be stated on good authority, occasionally on his own. In short, the subject is one with which he is fully conversant from every aspect.

During the month of January, 1962, Dr. Copeman paid a visit to the University of California at Los Angeles where he gave a series of lectures on the history of medicine. One of these dealt with the history of gout, and it was readily apparent that the speaker's grasp of his subject was such that it would have been a pity not to make it more widely known and at greater length than was possible in a single lecture. Despite his very busy professional life, Dr. Copeman generously yielded to entreaties to prepare a history *in extenso,* and as it has turned out he greatly enhanced the value of the original plan by including the history of gout's related complaints. Hence his book deals not only with the "queen of ailments" but with her sisters as well, in short the entire excruciating court of this realm.

C. D. O'MALLEY

Los Angeles, 25 July 1963

Preface

The influence of disease upon the history of mankind has been somewhat neglected by professional historians. History and disease, however, must be, like mind and body, inseparable, the one being inevitably influenced by the other.

Sydenham believed that gout was one of the earliest diseases to which flesh became heir when men began to participate in the luxuries of civilised life. It has certainly attracted the interest of medical historians from the time of ancient Greece, owing to its strikingly hereditary nature, to the sudden spectacular violence and periodicity of its attacks, and perhaps to its pleasing predilection for the great and wealthy—the *Morbus Dominorum*.

The vagaries of this disease have rendered leaders unpredictable and absented them without warning at critical periods of history. For this reason alone it may be thought that gout has been in the forefront of those diseases which have influenced the history of civilisation. That great statesman, Sir William Temple, wrote of the gout (1681):

> It generally falls upon persons engaged in Publick affairs and great employments upon whom . . . the Common Good, and the Service of their Countrie so much depends. . . . I have seen the Councils of a great countrie grow bold or timorous, and the pulse of Government beat high or low, according to the fits of gout or ill health of the Governors.

Gout has also been very much a part of the American scene since the sixteenth century. In 1592 Farfan published, in Mexico City, a medical treatise, twenty-one pages of which are devoted to the causes, symptoms, and treatment of gout; whilst Cadogan's classical work on gout reached seven editions during the colonial period in the British colonies of North America. Even the first Californian medical imprint, *Botica General*, Sonoma 1838, had a section on gout recommending: ". . . rub the affected area with puppy oil or warm bear's cub fat for several days. The patient will be permanently cured."

Its recurrent repercussions in the fields of literature, art, and drama have also been considerable. And, furthermore, the contemporary importance of this and other forms of arthritis and rheumatoid disease is tremendous, both in human suffering and wastage as well as in terms of cost. A recent Washington Committee on Productivity and Treatment estimated that the victims of these diseases themselves spend nearly a million dollars annually upon quack remedies alone!

The absence of a current historical survey of the gout and of its near relations, rheumatism and arthritis, thus seems curious, and the present volume is an attempt to fill this hiatus. It arose out of lectures delivered at the University of California, Los Angeles, at the invitation of Professor C. D. O'Malley, and the Woodward Lecture at Yale University, in 1962. To Professor O'Malley I am extremely indebted for much encouragement and help. My friend Dr. F. N. L. Poynter, of the Wellcome Historical Medical Library, and his staff have also, as usual, given me great assistance, especially with the illustrations, and Mr. L. M. Payne, the Librarian of the Royal College of Physicians, Mr. Philip Wade of the Royal Society of Medicine, and Dr. Francisco Guerra have afforded me considerable guidance. To Dr. George Spanopoulos of Athens I am grateful for drawing my attention to the gouty pedigree of the Medici, and to Miss Jessie Dobson for the loan of an illustration. I am indebted to the literary executors of the late E. F. Benson, and to the publishers Messrs. Longmans Green and Company, for permission to quote from his book *Final Edition* in the chapter on osteoarthritis. Mr. R. Y. Zachary, Los Angeles Editor of the University of California Press, has also been most kind and helpful.

London, 1963   W. S. C. COPEMAN

Contents

Illustrations

(following page 112)

CHAPTER I

A Synopsis of the Gout

The history of gout is an interesting one, and it has taken a long time to unfurl. Many of its individual episodes and personalities are dealt with in the following chapters. Some aspects of the story, however, remained unchanged for long periods, so it seems helpful to discuss these and others briefly in synoptic form to avoid the need for repetition later.

The Word

The word "gout" was not of medical origin, but was coined by the "barbarians" of Roman Europe and used as a lay colloquialism until the sixteenth century; perhaps it corresponded to the expression "the screws" now sometimes used to designate gout or rheumatism. It was derived directly from the Latin word *gutta* (a drop), in reference to the prevailing belief that an excess of one of the four humours, which in equilibrium were thought to maintain the body in health, would in certain circumstances drop or flow into a joint which had been previously weakened in some way, thus distending it and causing pain. The implications of this type of pathology were not, however, confined to joints, since such a flow of humours might obviously occur in any part of the body; and so we often meet with references to "gouty" migraine, diarrhoea, haemorrhoids, sciatica, and even gouty paralysis and epilepsy. The words "catarrh" and "rheumatism" were also used later to express the same conception of a flowing humour.

The first person who seems to have used the word gout in the modern sense to denote a painful periodical swelling of the big toe was the Dominican monk, Randolfus of Bocking, who was the domestic chaplain and biographer of Saint Richard, Bishop of Chichester (1197–1258). He recounted that he was a great sufferer with *gutta quam podagram vel arteticam vocant* (the gout which is called podagra or arthritis), and that he was completely cured by wearing a pair of his reverend superior's boots. It was thereafter widely and logically believed, as he tells us, that any sufferer privileged to place a gouty foot within the holy Bishop's boots would be ensured a speedy cure. The Bishop's effigy in stone still presides over the healing waters at Droitwich, the place of his birth. We also hear elsewhere in a contemporary account of the last Crusade (1270) that one of the leaders fell sick in Jerusalem of a "gote" in his knees and feet; whilst sufferers with the "gutta" were amongst those reported to have been miraculously cured at the tomb of St. Thomas à Becket in Canterbury about this time. According to Rodnan (1963) at least thirteen other saints and holy men gave evidence of similar therapeutic powers.

This specific use of the word was not, however, adopted throughout Europe until Guillaume de Baillou, whose name was Latinized as Ballonius, first clearly drew the distinction clinically between gout and rheumatism (1642), and Sydenham, a little later, made this separation final, as will be related below.

The Causes of Gout

Aretaeus the Cappadocian, a distinguished physician of the second century A.D., was uniquely modest in asserting of gout that "the basic cause of all this none but the gods can ever understand." Few others seriously doubted, until almost modern times, that the underlying cause of the disease was to be found in an imbalance or alteration of some sort in one or more of the four constituent humours of the body, as had been postulated by Galen. This unitarian theory seemed quite adequate to explain the observed facts. Aretaeus recognised that the tendency to gout might be inherited, and this he referred to as the gouty "diathesis." He also pointed out that "this disease remits sometimes for long periods . . . hence a person subject to the gout has been known to win the race in the Olympic Games during an interval of the disease."

Early in the sixteenth century in Europe, when chemistry was just beginning to emerge from alchemy, the eccentric Swiss peripatetic physician who called himself Paracelsus (1493–1541) sought to substitute a chemical for the humoral basis of both gout and the renal calculus. He thought that the cause of both might lie in the tendency of certain people's bodies to retain acrid substances which he believed were similar to those salts of tartar he had noticed deposited in wine barrels, and which in normal people would be excreted through the kidneys. This "theory of tartarous disease" seems to have been the first ever to postulate a chemical or metabolic aetiology for any disease.

This idea, of what we would now call an inborn error of metabolism, did not attract serious notice, however, until it was revived in rather different form during the eighteenth century, when William Cullen of Edinburgh (1710–1790), following the lead of Coste's *Traité Pratique sur la Goutte* (1757), endeavoured to correlate such a condition with certain recognisable external physical features. Cullen suggested that: "The gout attacks men especially of robust and large bodies, men of large heads . . . and men whose skins are covered with a thick

rete mucosum with coarse surface . . . especially men
of a choleric-sanguine type . . . (whose fathers had suffered)." It is, however, difficult, he continued, "rightly to
treat this matter with due precision." The idea received
support from William Cadogan (1771), who asked: "If
the features of the countenance, the outside of the body,
are often hereditary, why not also the inside?" We do not
seem to have advanced greatly beyond this point today.

Secondary, or aggravating factors, were also given due
importance in early times and were the object of considerable research. The Byzantine physician, Paul of
Aegina, recorded about A.D. 650 that mental stress could
prove a predisposing cause, declaring that "Sorrow, care,
watchfulness, and other passions of the mind may excite
an attack of this disorder." Much later, in the eighteenth
century, Sir Richard Blackmore, an English Royal Physician, also expressed the view that the cause of gout was
more metaphysical than physical, although he agreed
that a "scorbutic diathesis" might generally be an underlying factor. William Cadogan, commenting, said: "I
shall not enter deeply into the regions of metaphysical
conjecture . . . in guessing at the incomprehensible
union of body and soul and their mutual powers of acting
upon each other"; but it seemed to him that "vexation"
was one of the three great causes of gout, and indeed of
all chronic disease.

Hippocrates had recognised that excess in the consumption of certain wines could play a part in exacerbating, if
not actually causing, the disease, as would "venery." He
advised moderation in both. This viewpoint was widely
held, if not much acted upon, throughout the Middle
Ages and Renaissance. Alcohol was accorded an high
aetiological status by most physicians of the seventeenth,
eighteenth, and nineteenth centuries, although Syden-

ham's despairing aphorism was often quoted: "If you drink wine you get the gout; if you do not drink wine— the gout has you!" Contemporary views could perhaps be summarised in the picturesque phrase of a French physician who considered that "Gout is the afternoon of the pleasant day enjoyed by the sufferer's grandfather."

It was William Musgrave of Exeter who first (1703) reported that gonorrhoea and possibly other "fevers" could exacerbate the gout, and that lead could be its cause, especially in such occupations as painting and plumbing. This was later followed by two confirmatory reports from well-known physicians practising in Bath: Dr. William Falconer (1772), and Dr. Caleb H. Parry (1825). The latter was the first to describe the disease which now bears Graves's name, and was also the father of the famous arctic explorer, Sir William Parry.

In the nineteenth century both Jean Charcot and Sir Alfred Garrod published case reports showing this also. Cullen formed the opinion that the acute attack of gout did not depend upon the presence of impurity of any sort in the blood-stream. "Indeed," he wrote, "it attacks the very healthy, and so is extremely unlikely to be due to the presence of morbid matter in the system." He also thought that every case must be of hereditary origin because "as opposed to the rheumatism it seems to come on without other evident cause." It was only with Garrod's discovery (1848) that the circulating morbid matter which had been postulated by most of his predecessors was uric acid, that those further chemical studies could be initiated which led to our modern understanding of the disease.

Classification

Although the Aesculapian physicians regarded all affections of joints as being of the same basic gouty nature, evidence seems to show that Hippocrates himself recognised gout and rheumatic fever as being different syndromes. This distinction was forgotten by his successors, however, until halfway through the sixteenth century, although there is some reason to believe that Soranus of Ephesus, a physician of the second century A.D. also distinguished between gout and other forms of adult arthritis, a matter which will be referred to in a later chapter. Sydenham, commenting upon this (1683) dryly remarked: "Doubtless gout and rheumatism were often confounded by the ancient Greek physicians; a point which is still equally applicable to the pundits of our present day."

Thus, from the later Greek writings onwards, the generic term used was "arthritis," and usually its varieties were merely classified upon an anatomical plan: podagra when it affected the foot, chiagra the hand, gonagra the knee, and so on throughout the joints of the body. This remained the popular arrangement for the next thousand years. Henry VIII's physician, Andrew Boorde (1490–1549), deplored the habit of giving the name arthritis to the affections of all the joints "whether the pain arise from a rheumatic inflammation or a gouty humor." He described four types of gout, namely chiagra, of hands, fingers, and arms; podagra, of the feet, toes, and legs; "Goute arterycke, which involves jointes elsewhere"; and sciatica. He warned that "all jointe illnesses are not the goute." In reply to criticism levelled at him for doubting in some respects the authority of Galen, he remarked very sensibly that: "It is extremely difficult for a physician who puts too much trust in what he reads to form a proper decision from what he sees."

The only important new idea was that proposed by Rufus of Ephesus, later amplified by Paul of Aegina, which introduced the concept of visceral or "metastatic" gout, whereby the disease might leave the joints and attack the chief internal organs, sometimes with fatal results. The frequent association of gout with stone in the kidney or bladder was also recognised and recorded at this time. The great French Renaissance physician, Jean Fernel (1497–1558), and Jerome Cardan (1501–1576), a learned and fashionable physician of Pavia whose consulting practice extended as far as Scotland, independently revived the long-forgotten Hippocratic belief that rheumatic fever was an entity separate from podagra. Cardan was the first to point out the predominantly pediatric association of rheumatic fever, when he wrote: "The Morbus Articularis and the podagra are not the same. I have seen many children suffering with arthritis, but never with podagra; and I cannot recollect ever having justly read of one." He observed also that relapses of rheumatic arthritis, unlike those of podagra, tended to occur only in the presence of a fever. This important distinction was re-emphasised by the posthumous publication of Baillou's *Liber de Rhumatismo* (1642), but was not completely accepted by the profession until Sydenham (1683) further elucidated the distinction, dividing gout, of which he had a long, personal experience, into the acute and chronic varieties, and describing rheumatic fever for the first time with accuracy.

With the eighteenth century came the fashion, started in botany by Linnaeus, for evolving "systems" of classification, and articular rheumatic disease received considerable attention from such leaders of the profession in Europe as Hermann Boerhaave, William Cullen, William Musgrave, George Cheyne, Richard Mead, Van Swieten, Friedrich Hoffmann, William Cadogan, and William Heberden.

Although it was Linnaeus who first established the vogue for classification, it was his friend, the Frenchman

François de Sauvages (1706–1767), who, in his *Nosologia Methodica*, published in Amsterdam in 1763, made the first serious attempt to classify the articular diseases. Gout he subdivided into no fewer than fourteen varieties, although as Scudamore later pointed out, he only did this "out of those modifications which the disease sometimes assumes by combination with other diseases, or by the influence of the season of the year." Sauvages, following Sydenham, recognised some types as being provoked by physical or mental stress, and some by "fevers and other causes."

William Cullen proposed a slightly simpler general classification in his *Synopsis Nosologiae Methodicae* (1769), in which all diseases were divided into four main groups: the fevers, the nervous diseases, local diseases, and "the cachexiae, or diseases resulting from a bad habit of body." It was in this last category that he placed all the rheumatic diseases and their subdivisions, including gout, which he, like his master Boerhaave, always referred to as podagra. In Cullen's system "gout is of the *Species Idiopathica* and is subdivided into four categories: first the Regular; then the Irregular," which he defined as "Whatever symptoms we can perceive to be connected with the disposition which produces the inflammatory affection of the joints, but without being present at the same time." It was this latter type that William Musgrave (1703), and later Cheyne (1720), termed "Anomalous" gout. This category Cullen further subdivided into the "Atonic," which afflicted the stomach and gastrointestinal tract, and the "Retrocedent," in which joint pain became suddenly transferred to some internal organ.

A variant of this was the "Misplaced" type, in which the gouty lesion was internal from the beginning. Cullen quoted, for example, those chronic cases in which the joint pains would often alternate with affections of the stomach or other internal parts, what he called "a sort of reciprocal sympathetic action." Scudamore (1816) rightly found this conception to be "very inaccurate in theory and practice; it gives us unbounded latitude to call every disease occurring in a gouty individual as *disguised gout* arising out of this." The terms "gouty eczema" and "gouty stomach" are still not unknown today.

Pathology

It was only subsequent to the reintroduction of sound observational medicine by Sydenham that the pathology of gout began to arouse real interest. This was stimulated by the general use of the microscope in the latter eighteenth century, and the pathology of gout was first described systematically by the Italian, Giovanni Battista Morgagni (1682–1771), and by Alexander Monro *Secundus* (1733–1817) in Edinburgh. Bichat, the father of French scientific medicine, added to this study, and demonstrated the different post-mortem appearances in gout and rheumatism in his great work, *Anatomie Pathologique* (1825), which first supplied a fully objective basis for the study of disease.

The first step towards an accurate metabolic conception was taken by the Swedish apothecary, Karl Wilhelm Scheele (1742–1786), who conducted what we should now term basic chemical research in the kitchen of his herb shop after business hours. In 1776, unaided, he discovered uric acid, which he named "Lithic acid," and he was able ten years later to demonstrate its presence as a normal constituent in human urine. He died at the early age of forty-four years, it is said of rheumatism.

Later W. H. Wollaston (1766–1828), F.R.S., the great chemist, Fellow of Caius College, Cambridge, and nephew of Dr. Heberden, similarly examined a gouty tophus which he picked out of his own ear for this purpose, and showed that this also was composed of sodium urate.

Sir Alfred Garrod (1819–1907) first demonstrated that it was this substance which constituted the "morbid circulating matter" in the blood in cases of gout (1848). His book, *The Nature and Treatment of Gout and Gouty Arthritis*, described his simple but effective "thread test," whereby uric acid could be precipitated in crystalline form and the diagnosis of gout be thus confirmed by the physician at the patient's bedside; surely one of the first clinical diagnostic tests ever to be devised.

It was the monumental work of the German chemist, Emil Fischer (1852–1919), which first established the relationship of uric acid to purine protein bodies. He worked out the family tree of gout and showed that the purine nucleus was the common ancestor of all the metabolic products of the disease. In this way he laid the foundations of our present understanding of the metabolism of gout.

The anatomical, pathological, and descriptive work of Todd, Bichat, Garrod, and the other scientific physicians of the nineteenth century was the fulfillment of that of Morgagni and his school, and established our basic knowledge on firm foundations. In spite of all this new work, however, old ideas died hard, and the profession was reluctant until our own time to recognise gout as a separate and specific biochemical disorder, and to relinquish the idea of it having a common humoral "diathesis" causing many and varied disorders throughout the body. Since then we have learnt but little more of the fundamental mechanism of gout, although we have made considerable advances in the micro-methods of blood analysis, and, largely as the result of this, in the therapeutic field. Even in this twentieth century, however, gout has still not yielded up its final secrets.

Prognosis

With regard to the prognosis of the disease, Hippocrates, some five centuries before Christ, said that those affected with the gout "who are aged and have tophi in their joints, and those who have led a hard life and whose bowels are constipated, are beyond the power of medicine to cure. . . . Persons under other circumstances may be cured by a skilfull physician." This wide view of the prognosis of the disease remained almost unchanged until comparatively modern times. Since the introduction of modern uricosuric preparations, however, the future of the gouty patient can generally be considered fairly bright.

Treatment

The general plan of treatment advocated by the ancients, based as it was upon the humoral theory of disease, remained remarkably constant throughout the Greek, Roman, Byzantine, Moslem, and Mediaeval periods. The object was to get rid of the offending matter from the system by all available routes. Once this had been accomplished, according to Hippocrates, the body would act as its own physician. The methods employed were, therefore, bleeding and blistering, sweating, purging with scammony, white hellebore, or other herbal cathartics, and the administration of emetics and diuretics. Hippocrates himself tended to favour the less violent types of treatment, and in his empirical approach he would have agreed with the general advice given by St. Paul in another connection: to "prove all things; hold fast that which is good."

The Greeks' frequent use of hermodactyl, a close relation of *Colchicum autumnale*, was probably not recognised by them as specific therapy, this plant being normally administered merely as a drastic purge. It was only later noticed by some physicians, notably by Alexander of Tralles (A.D. 525–605), that its effect was of a more direct nature. This matter is more fully discussed in Chapter III.

From earliest times, and through the Middle Ages, great importance was always placed upon a regime of abstinence in diet and wine, especially at the commencement of an attack. This principle was recognised by Thomas Cogan when he wrote in 1584 that "poore men who cannot eate but seldome have it." The principle—rather than the practice—remains today. Healthy sleep was encouraged by all means, including moderate regular exercise; and excess in "venery in all its forms" was to be avoided. Galen advocated in addition a prophylactic course of bleeding and purging to be carried out in spring and late summer. All these practices were combined by the nineteenth century in the regime at "watering places" such as Wiesbaden and Aix which sprang up all over Europe and which it became fashionable to visit in order "to take the cure."

Many famous physicians throughout the ages had their own special mixtures, cordials, elixirs, or "specifics," but most of these appear to have been simple and harmless herbal concoctions whose efficacy may have owed more to the personality and fame of the prescriber than to the ingredients. The "Gout Cordial" of Boerhaave (1728), for instance, consisted of an equal mixture of rhubarb, senna, extract of licorice, and aromatics, digested in proof spirit. This continued to be advocated by Cullen, and was used until well into the nineteenth century. Some of the "specifics" introduced with fraudulent intent by quacks will be referred to in later chapters. Thus the medicinal treatment of gout remained unoriginal until the re-introduction of colchicum towards the beginning of the nineteenth century, after which a spate of "secret" remedies containing this drug appeared upon the markets of Europe. The uricosuric drugs were introduced during the present century and marked a great step forwards.

Local applications have been varied: fermentations both hot and cold, emollient ointments, counter-irritation by means of the cautery or burning flax, scarification by knife and blister, hot sand, and saline and mineral-water baths; and sometimes light friction of the affected joints with salt and oil. There was, however, always a school of thought which judged it to be dangerous to employ local measures of any sort, at any rate during the acute attack, in case they should interfere with nature's own efforts to expel the peccant humour, which seemed to them to be the purpose of the acute attacks.

Most physicians during the seventeenth and eighteenth centuries greatly over-treated their patients with the gross and debilitating methods at their disposal. Sydenham's was the first influential voice since Greek times to preach unfashionable moderation; and subsequently both Boerhaave's and Cullen's practice followed closely that of their great predecessor.

In addition, the latter two advocated a whey or milk diet and regular horseback riding, or if that were impossible, then "frequent riding in a coach"—coaches had no springs in those days! This latter advice was later reiterated by both Scudamore and Garrod, who considered the effect of exercise to be almost specific in clearing up the after-effects of an acute attack.

Views on bleeding varied greatly through the ages.

Until the time of Sydenham it had been widely advocated and extensively used. The principal points of controversy had been whether it should be carried out on the side of the body opposite the lesion (in the fashion of the Moslems), or on the side near the joint, or even in another limb; also whether the lancet or the leech was the preferable instrument. "Wet cupping" was introduced as an additional refinement towards the end of the eighteenth century. Sydenham, with considerable originality for his time, declared himself as being normally against the whole procedure. Nevertheless he declared that "If the patient be young, and have drunk hard, blood may be drawn at the beginning of the fit. If, however, it be continued during the following attacks gout will take up its quarters, even in a young subject; and its Empire will be no Government but a Tyranny." The great French surgeon, Ambroise Paré, considered, however, that "It is hardly possible to be too drastic," particularly if permanent establishment of the disease was to be thwarted. Well into the nineteenth century Gairdner (1849) wrote in favour of small, repeated bleedings: "It is with me no manner of doubt but of absolute certainty that in plethoric individuals much suffering may be saved, and no injury done." Garrod himself still used it occasionally in early cases who were otherwise healthy, but he was against the local use of leeches or blisters to affected joints as slow-healing sores so often resulted. Therapeutic bleeding has been used in the treatment of many gouty patients who are still living.

With regard to purging, a similar variation of opinion had existed even amongst the Greeks, and considerable variety and ingenuity in the compounding of purgative prescriptions was shown from Roman times onwards. Polypharmacy was the rule during the Middle Ages and combinations of many drastic cathartics were usual. A prescription which became so popular throughout Europe that its official pharmacopoeial name was "Pilulae sine quibus esse nolo" (pills without which I would not wish to be), contained aloes, scammony, senna, colocynth, and rhubarb, and purported to give "relief to a burdened brain by purging phlegm"—surely an understatement of fact. The sceptical Culpeper, in his *London Dispensatory Further Adorned* (1679) said of this famous remedy: "I had rather let them alone than take them. I doubt they were mistaken, it should have been 'Pilulae sine quibus esse *volo*.' "

Perhaps the most momentous, although fortuitous, landmark in the early history of gout was Sydenham's well-known personal antagonism to purgation, as this automatically also banished the use of colchicum, which was still a frequent constituent of many cathartic prescriptions. His theoretical objection to purgings was based upon Galen's view that "Nature seems to have the prerogative to expel the peccant matter according to its own method." "Sure I am," Sydenham wrote, "that all purging, mild or sharp, intended to relieve the joints, is injurious, whether it be during a fit to diminish the peccant matter, at the end to dissipate its remnants, or during an intermission to guard against the occurrence of one." But he also had personal experience and related that: "From myself and others I have learnt that purges bring on what they were meant to keep off." As the result Europe had to wait two hundred years for the benefit of the re-introduction of colchicum as treatment for acute gout.

Both Richard Mead and Boerhaave shared this reluctance to purge, although they would sometimes order small doses of Glauber's salt, a recent introduction from the continent. Purgation was restored to fashionable favour by Sir Charles Scudamore in the eighteen-twenties.

He advocated a formidable-sounding combination of calomel, antimony, and compound extract of colocynth, repeating it nightly or every second day for a time. He said that he would often add to this a draught of magnesium sulphate and extract of colchicum—our forefathers were a sturdy breed.

The clyster, a refinement which was popular prior to and during the eighteenth century, was a large form of enema syringe made out of a pig's bladder, with which various mixtures—which generally contained honey—were injected for the purpose of clearing the lower bowel of its "excrementous residuum."

All these rather fierce methods of treatment received a temporary setback when Dr. William Cadogan (1711–1799) published his best-selling book, *A Dissertation on the Gout and on All Chronic Diseases* (1771), which he dedicated "to all invalids." In it, he refuted specific treatment and, with great originality as was then thought, advocated a permanently temperate way of life. He wrote: "How ill can vomiting, bleeding and purging supply the place of temperance; cordials and opium of peace of mind? . . . It is the constant course of life which we lead, what we do, or neglect to do habitually that, if right, establishes our health; if wrong, makes us invalids for life." Nevertheless he later relented somewhat and said that: "I think the causes may be very fairly reduced to these three: Indolence, Intemperance and Vexation. . . . It is by their own fault that they are ill. Nonetheless medical treatment *can* do good." Dr. Samuel Johnson was asked his opinion of this work by Boswell, and thought that: " 'Tis a good book in general, Sir, but a foolish one as to particulars." No doubt this was because for his own gout Johnson preferred and practised drastic treatment which included enormous doses of Dr. James's powder of antimony, such as were supposed to have killed his friend, Oliver Goldsmith; he taunted Dr. William Heberden, who tried to dissuade him from this, with the title of "Dr. Timidorum Timidissimus." The other celebrated advocate of "the good temperate life" in the management of gout at this time was Dr. George Cheyne of Bath (1671–1743), a pupil of Pitcairn, who wrote on similar lines but, although himself a *bon viveur*, went so far as to recommend strict vegetarianism in certain cases.

In medicinal treatment it was the same with anodynes. Hippocrates had warned against them, and Sydenham avoided their use when he could. Cullen wrote: "Whilst opiates give the most certain relief from pain, yet when given in the beginning of a gouty paroxysm they cause it to return later with even greater volume." Garrod himself withheld them if possible, owing to "their baneful influence upon the secreting organs," but if pressed he would prescribe a little Dover's powder (compound powder of ipecacuanha), or occasionally some henbane or belladonna.

About 1780 a French regimental officer, M. Nicholas Husson, discovered a method of extracting and standardising the potency of the autumn crocus (*Colchicum autumnale*), of which the value had earlier been rediscovered but ineffectively publicised by Von Stoerk in Vienna. Husson was able to preserve its effectiveness for long periods and patented and advertised it extensively as the secret "specific," *L'Eau d'Husson,* which had immediate, enormous success throughout Europe. Its active principle was identified as colchicum in 1814, and this turned the attention of the new medical chemists not only to the study of colchicum, but to the pathology and biochemistry of gout generally.

Tophi

"Those little chalky excrescences not unlike crabs' eyes," as Sydenham had called them, were well recognised and described as a feature of gout by all the ancient writers. But it is a curious fact, noted by Delpeuch, that their well-observed occurrence in the ears of gouty patients received no published notice until the sixteenth century. Soranus of Ephesus, writing during the second century A.D., said in the course of his excellent description of the gout: "Then stones develop that disorganise the joints and distend the skin. These may burst through and jut out. They can be removed surgically, or upon their early appearance may be merely lifted out with a spoon-shaped instrument, though later they will grow again." His colleague, Rufus of Ephesus, mentions that he had occasionally seen them dissolve during the course of treatment. The majority of other Greek writers preferred to leave them *in situ* if they did not respond to simple heat and poultices. Occasionally they would endeavour to dissolve them away with a paste of quicklime and nitre in lard, but we hear little of this sort of approach through the Middle Ages.

With the dawn of chemistry in the eighteenth century it was proposed by Boerhaave, who believed the tophi to be composed of true chalk, that they should be dissolved away by the frequent application of a few drops of hydrochloric acid in turpentine. His pupil, Van Swieten, claimed good results by the use of a compound made by heating crude tartar with a solution of quicklime in water, and reported that they would often disappear within a few days.

In the nineteenth century Sir Charles Scudamore sometimes used to attempt to dissolve them with a solution of

potash, whilst his successor, Sir Alfred Garrod, thought
that this end could sometimes be achieved with the use
of lithia. It is only during the last few years that efficient
uricosuric agents have been devised by which, if the level
of uric acid in the blood can be controlled, the tophi
will also dissolve and often ultimately disappear.

Summary

It is of interest to the medical historian to remark that
practically all the beliefs and therapeutic methods prior
to our own time which have been briefly noted above
had their origin in Greek times and were passed down
basically unchanged until the opening of the nineteenth
century. With the exception of emetics all these methods
appear to have had the sanction of the "High-Priest of
Gout" Sir Alfred Garrod, who died as recently as 1907.

It was with the discovery of the uricosuric substances
that the modern conception of long-term treatment
started. These drugs are able to increase the excretion
of uric acid from the body and so lower its level in the
blood-stream. The first of these was cinchophen (atophan)
whose dangerous side effects tended to negate its therapeutic value. Its use led, however, to the present strategy
whereby acute attacks of gout are controlled with alkaloid
colchicine or phenylbutazone, together with a moderate
dietetic regime; and long-term "interval treatment" by
means of a uricosuric is maintained with the idea of
gradually preventing the occurrence of further acute episodes altogether. The modern type of uricosuric drugs
was discovered only about fifteen years ago, almost by
accident arising out of the war-time penicillin research.

With our newly established power of controlling gout,
its original "status" has suffered. It had previously seemed
some compensation for its ravages that the victims it

chose were amongst the highest in all countries. The *Times* commented in 1900 "The common cold is well named—but the gout seems instantly to raise the patient's social status." Only this year the journal *Punch* wrote, however, that "in keeping with the spirit of more democratic times gout is becoming less upper-class and is now open to all . . . it is ridiculous that a man should be barred from enjoying gout because he went to the wrong school." However, it has perhaps always been commoner than has been recognised. It was Hench who only a few years ago drew attention to the high proportion of un-diagnosed examples in the United States in an article he rightly entitled "Gout—the Forgotten Disease."

CHAPTER II

Gout in the Earliest Times

Hippocrates and His Followers

The oldest medical textbook which we possess is made up of those excellent treatises known as the works of Hippocrates. These seem to date from about the fifth century B.C., and show a good practical knowledge of disease based upon direct clinical observations.

Hippocrates as a person is a somewhat nebulous figure, although he is thought by some to have been a consultant physician and teacher at the Temple of Healing on the Greek island of Cos, where his father, a descendant of the deified physician, Aesculapius, had also practised. In middle life Hippocrates spent a period in Macedonia as court physician to the King, whom he is said to have cured of "the love-sickness" as a young prince. He was also called to Athens at the time of the great plague, which he is reported to have extinguished by means of strategically placed bonfires. The great plane tree under which he is said to have given his medical lectures can still be seen at Cos and has healthy descendants in many parts of the world.

His contemporaries constituted perhaps the most remarkable galaxy of genius ever known. They included Pericles, the statesman and builder of the Acropolis; the poets and playwrights, Aeschylus, Sophocles, Euripides, Aristophanes, and Pindar, whose nephew was one of Hippocrates' students; the philosopher, Socrates, with his disciples, Plato and Xenophon; the venerable father of history, Herodotus, with his youthful rival, Thucydides; and the sculptor, Phidias.

Hippocrates' writings are free of the prevailing superstitions which associated the cause of disease with divine wrath for sin and much of therapy with magic. He observed objectively and collected clinical facts, and in this way compiled what he rightly referred to as the Natural History of Disease. Thus he justified his title as the "Father of Medicine" in its modern connotation.

In surgical practice he seems to have been a bold operator, opening the chest for pleural infections and often trephining the skull for what sound to us like relatively minor injuries and diseases.

Therapeutically he advocated common sense: dietetics, and the use of all empirically proved remedies if used "in such a way as to do good, or at least to do no harm."

Hippocrates regarded gout as being the result of an excessive accumulation of one of the bodily humours, probably phlegm, which distended the affected joint painfully. This might result from sexual excess, or too rich a diet together with a sedentary life. Much later Galen, in his commentary on the *Aphorisms,* added an hereditary factor, and noted that those who inherited gout tended to suffer more severely than those who acquired it. Many of the heroes of Greek mythology are said to have suffered with the gout. Amongst these we hear of King Priam of Troy, Achilles, Bellepheron who died of it, and Oedipus, King of Thebes.

The three famous surviving *Aphorisms* of Hippocrates which refer to gout (nos. 28, 29, and 30) have often been quoted but may be repeated:

First: "Eunuchs do not take the gout, nor become bald." Galen, in his later commentary, whilst agreeing that this was basically true, said that in this time, however, such was their indolence and viciousness that they occasionally did so.

Second: "A woman does not take the gout unless her menses be stopped." Here again Galen said that in his time younger women, from an excess of modern luxury in contrast to the austere life that had been led under the Republic, had become subject to gout. Seneca, also discussing the luxury and vice of the Empire, affirmed the same: "The nature of women is not altered since the days of the Republic, but their manner of living. In this age women rival men in every kind of lasciviousness . . . why need we then be surprised at seeing so many of the female sex afflicted with the gout?" Nonetheless he deplored "this setback to the authority of the physicians who had always asserted their little likelihood to this disease." He later referred to the pedigree of the disease as being the rosy daughter of the long line of Bacchus and Venus: "Bacchus pater, Venus mater, et Ira obstetrix Arthritidis."

Lastly: "A young man does not take the gout until he indulges in coitus." By this Hippocrates probably meant before the age of puberty.

This evident sex linkage with male virility, here and elsewhere so frequently emphasised by the highest authority, underlay aetiological thinking until comparatively modern times, and we even find castration seriously proposed as a cure for chronic sufferers as late as the eighteenth century.

Hippocrates marked the periodicity of the attacks, saying (Aphorism 55): "For the most part gouty affections rankle in the Spring and in the Autumn." He had also remarked earlier, and less specifically, that amongst the diseases of the spring are the arthritic diseases. Later commentators, notably Celsus, explained the autumn exacerbation as being nature's effort to expel to the extremities those peccant humours which had accumulated in the body during the heat of the summer.

There can be very little doubt that Hippocrates was able to distinguish between acute gout and acute rheumatism, which he termed arthritis. In his *Affections of the Parts* he compared them. "Podagra," he said, "is the most violent of all joint affections, it lasts long, and becomes chronic. . . . The pain may remain fixed in the great toes . . . it is not fatal." Later he declared: "In arthritis fever comes on, acute pain affects the joints of the body, and the pains which vary between mild and severe flit from joint to joint; it is of short duration, and often very acute, but not mortal. It attacks the young more frequently than the old."

Hippocrates and his Greek followers believed in the efficacy of diet in the control of gout, emphasising not only the types of food to be taken or avoided, but also the best methods of preparing them—"whereby the humours may be kept in healthy balance and disease obviated." He discussed the nature of wines fully, and he did not forbid the use of them entirely, particularly for elderly patients. He strongly advocated the use of a form of barley water called ptisan, however, of which Sydenham much later also greatly approved.

Hippocrates was occasionally prepared to get tough with intractable cases of chronic gout by the use of heroic doses of the powerful purgative, white hellebore (*Veratrum album*) since, as he pointed out, "the best natural relief for this disease is an attack of dysentery."

Of the local treatment of chronic gouty joints he remarked: "This is a long, painful, but not a mortal illness; if the pain still continue, burn the veins above the joints with raw flax." It is interesting to note that this method of counter-irritation was introduced into England during the eighteenth century from the East Indies, using a form of cotton plant named moxa.

Somewhere between the time of Hippocrates and the foundation of the Roman Empire, the Old Testament canon and the laws of the Prophets were written in the Middle East. In these we find a description of the ritual of consecration for the Jewish priesthood. C. J. Brim, in his *Medicine in the Bible* (1936), suggests that part of this was an allusion to the gout, which was a common affliction of the Semitic race. The blood of the sacrificial ram was placed on the priest's great toe, the base of the thumb, and on the ears, the favourite sites for the disease. All wine drinking was strictly forbidden; and in allusion perhaps to gout's hereditary nature all the sons of Aaron were also prophylactically exposed to this ritual. The reason for all this perhaps becomes clearer when we read in the Talmud the opinion of the rabbis that the cause of most of their common diseases at this early period in history could be ascribed to a sedentary life, laziness, over-eating and drinking.

The Romans and Byzantines

In time the political and intellectual centre of the Western world shifted from Greece, *via* Alexandria, to Rome. Prior to this the Romans appear to have paid very little serious attention either to the art of medicine or to disease itself. There was no native school of physicians before the Greeks came, although intelligent slaves were trained as medical orderlies and masseurs. According to the Elder Pliny, who was a dedicated nationalist, there had been no gout in Italy, although rheumatic fever

seems to have been indigenous, and as proof that gout
was an unwelcome and novel Greek import he cited the
fact that there was no Latin name for it.

Although the Romans initiated nothing in medicine
they were great classifiers and codifiers. The most celebrated of these contemporary medical encyclopoedias was
that of Celsus.

Celsus (25 B.C.–A.D. 50) was not a physician but a well-
educated country gentleman who, whilst living quietly
on his estate near Rome in his later years, produced his
great literary labour of love in eight books entitled *De re
Medicina*, in which he summarised all contemporary
knowledge of human and veterinary medicine. Reflecting
the views of his time he recognised one basic affection of
the joints which he termed "arthritis," adapting the more
precise terminology of the disease to its local site. Arthritis, podagra, chiagra, and so forth, were therefore
considered to be scientifically interchangeable terms in
his writings.

He stressed the importance of a regulated manner of
living, the avoidance of corpulence, and the need for
moderate regular exercise—none of these being inherent
in the contemporary Roman way of life; indeed, as he
points out, practically every one of the Roman emperors
had suffered with gout, "whether of their own fault or
that of their progenitors I know not." The Consul
Agrippa endured three acute attacks and committed suicide at the onset of his fourth rather than endure it.
Celsus advocated moderate bleeding from a vein at the
commencement of an acute attack of gout, as he claimed
to have noticed that this procedure had the effect of
causing the first affected joints to remain free of pain

until the next annual recurrence of the disease—and in some cases even for life.

It was Celsus who perpetuated doubts, which persisted until the last century, regarding the wisdom of external local treatment to affected joints. He granted that warm applications might sometimes be permissible, according to the degree of inflammation present; but he enjoined the greatest caution with regard to cold, believing that this might lower the resistance of the joint, and so frustrate nature's efforts to dispel the disease through the medium of the acute attack, thus driving it inwards again towards more vital organs. The great Moslem physician, Avicenna, writing in the eleventh century, drew attention to the importance of this belief, which became the academic view throughout Mediaeval Europe. As a compromise he suggested that intractable joints might be lightly cauterised with a hot iron through a layer of salt and oil.

The subject of gout exercised a fascination for many of the chief literary figures of the Imperial Roman period, most of whom do not appear to have formed a very high opinion of the therapeutic results attained by their medical colleagues. These included Virgil, Martial, and Ovid. The last agreed in verse with the view of Hippocrates: *Tollere nodosam nescit medicina podagram* (Physicke cannot the knotty [tophaceous] goute well heale); and in his *Epistle to Pontus* he also stated authoritatively that no cure could be expected where time and tophi were in command. Pliny and Seneca made frequent allusions to podagra, relating its origins to the riotous living which was fashionable at this period. Seneca, in his ninety-fifth Epistle, voiced the cynical assumption that it would never be amenable to the treatment of physicians, and advised a stoical indifference to its present agonies.

The "theme song" of one of Lucian's comic plays is addressed to chronic sufferers and may be loosely translated as follows:

> Celebrate with hymns your invisible goddess Podagra—
> Hope always that your long, long sufferings will serve you
>   for consolation,
> Have joyful hearts; forget your agony.
> Give yourselves over to laughter and pleasure
> —as you've got it for keeps!

Lucian's comic "tragedies," the *Tragopodagra* and the *Ocypus*, show a remarkable medical knowledge of the disease, both subjectively and objectively, to such an extent that it has been generally assumed that he himself was a sufferer. His descriptions were considered by Van Swieten (English edition 1760) to be of such accuracy that he quotes Lucian's verses no less than forty times during the course of his commentary on the aphorisms of Boerhaave on this subject. The "star" of Lucian's play, *Tragopodagra*, is the "Demon Goddess Podagra." "Who does not know me? Gout, the unconquered Goddess of all earthly ills! Whom neither Apollo, doctor of all Gods celestial, nor the son of Apollo, the most learned Aesculapius, is able to expel." Her boast as she retires in her triumphant finale, having crippled all the doctors sent from earth to overcome her, is: "Thus all those who use powerful remedies, daring to fight determinedly against me, shall only encounter my greater rage, and shall themselves fall—as to the others I shall be sweet and clement." The text of this play reveals in succinct form the complete armamentarium at the disposal of the physician called upon to treat gout "determinedly" during the second century after Christ. It was remarkably wide and mostly extremely unpleasant. Remedies included raw toad and human excrement in addition to the more widely accepted herbal and mineral medicaments.

The next great physician of antiquity who wrote extensively on gout was Soranus of Ephesus (A.D. 98–138), who practised successfully in Rome under the emperors Trajan and Hadrian. His original works have been lost, but a Latin translation of these by a fifth-century physician, Caelius Aurelianus, was an important factor in preserving the tradition of Greek medical thought through the Middle Ages in Europe. In this work we can recognise that Soranus was a wise and humane physician of good sense and broad philosophical and historical interests. His books, *On Acute and Chronic Diseases*, include good sections on disease of the joints, and also on sciatica and lumbago, which latter he terms psoitis. It seems also evident that he, like Hippocrates, distinguished between gout and general acute polyarthritis. Moreover, being of what was known as the Dogmatic School, he did not subscribe to the humoral hypothesis and so was prepared to think that the aetiology and pathology of the two conditions might be different, although he did not differentiate their treatment.

His senior colleague, Rufus of Ephesus, who tells us that he himself was a victim of gout, initiated in the several works he wrote on this subject the conception of visceral or "metastatic" gout. He taught that the internal organs could become affected mortally by the gouty humour being driven inwards suddenly as the result of too-rapid cooling of the affected joints; or alternately as the result of stopping a course of internal treatment too abruptly. He said: "Such sudden revulsion of the humours from the joints will provoke pulmonary or cerebral complications, and in the same way failure of the renal and intestinal functions may produce a fatal result, generally preceded by convulsions and coma." He propounded the curious therapeutic axiom that when gout was confined to the feet, the patient should be ordered emetic treatment, but if it affected the upper limbs then purgatives, principally colocynth, should be prescribed. His works were greatly plagiarised by his successors, and throughout the Middle Ages many empirical "cures" were ascribed to his authority.

In the second century A.D., a very important period in the history of medicine, the major physicians were Galen and Aretaeus the Cappadocian. Within their extensive works the Hippocratic system of medicine was finally merged with the humoral hypothesis and rendered so rigid and precise that clinicians were unfortunately diverted from further original thought or clinical observation until the time of the European Renaissance. In spite of the fact that these two eminent practitioners were contemporaries no reference is found of either to the other in their voluminous writings. Adams, the translator of Aretaeus, rather naively wondered whether this might be considered "to denote a concealed feeling of rivalry?"

Galen (A.D. 130–200) was born at Pergamon in Asia Minor where he became medical officer to the Imperial training school for gladiators. This post gave him great experience in traumatic surgery and anatomy prior to his move to Rome, which he undertook at the request of the Emperor Marcus Aurelius, whose personal physician he became. He was a successful doctor, a great experimentalist, and was the author of more than eighty treatises which still exist, on various aspects of medicine, anatomy, physiology, and surgery. He appears to have been sympathetic to Christianity, although never converted. He died whilst on vacation in Sicily at the age of seventy, as the result, according to one of his colleagues, of taking his own remedies.

Galen was Hippocrates' greatest follower and admirer. What the Master had begun he was to bring to the greatest possible perfection. The merest glance through his writings will show that he was a true and brilliant scientist who advanced medical knowledge on the basis of the experimental method. It was not his fault that his works appeared to his successors to have been so profound that no modification seemed necessary during the next thousand years; but it is ironical that such a man should, as the result, have initiated the dark ages of medical decadence. His style was more verbose and philosophical than was that of Hippocrates, and his therapeutic approach was more violent as befitted the sophisticated taste of the inhabitants of the busy centre of the Western world in which he practised and wrote.

It is evident from his works that Galen was not a modest man. He was, however, a dynamic seeker after true knowledge and he would have deplored the fact that his works produced a static cult.

At this time the rheumatic diseases were still grouped under the single heading of "arthritis" and named according to the part of the body chiefly affected. The differentiation between gout and rheumatic fever which Hippocrates had observed was evidently much less clearly recognised by his followers. In the case of podagra Galen deviated from the hypothesis of general humoral imbalance in believing that the cause of this disease lay in an unnatural accumulation of humours in the affected part only, and that tophi were the resulting local concretions which had oozed out of the joint.

Therapeutically he advocated a similar dietetic regime to that advised by Hippocrates, but added also prophy-

lactic bleeding or purging of known sufferers every spring
unless already crippled. He felt that diet was the key
factor influencing health and disease, and that the indications varied according to the type of disease and the
temperament of each patient, although he laid down general rules based upon the humoral hypothesis. These
comprised the use of plain, easily digested food: "Barley bread is a very excellent thing, and a sausage in
due season; and a little cabbage half boiled, with a soup
of mixed vegetables." He also suggested as permissible,
parsnips, "sea foods" such as oyster, limpet, and sea-
urchin soup, but only "such fishes as inhabit rocky
places." Of land animals he favoured chiefly mutton, goat,
hares, and the wild boar, but strictly forbade pork; "and
of winged beasts all sorts of partridge, small birds, wood
pigeon and domestic pigeon." Fruits should be taken
only during the summer months and sparingly. A sea
voyage in the spring can be very beneficial also, he said—
no doubt this would have involved considerable dietetic
restriction in those days, alternating with periods of
emesis. As regards medicinal treatment Galen was unoriginal and something of a sceptic. He believed that the
more violent and even dangerous methods shunned by
Hippocrates might be justified for intractable gout if
the patient wished it.

Although in general principles against the imbibing
of alcohol by the gouty, Sabine wine found in Galen an
advocate, particularly for the elderly sufferer, but he
recommended the addition to every draught of some
sprigs of rock parsley "which contains a diuretic principle
which is desirable for the arthritis; and I do not forbid
old men to use even the sweet wines in the gout if there
is a suspicion of calculus in the kidneys."

Of Aretaeus the Cappadocian (fl. A.D. 135) little seems

to be known. From the epithet, "the Cappadocian," with which his name is always associated, it is to be assumed that he was born in Asia Minor, although it seems from references in his works that he must have spent most of his life, like Galen, in Rome. His description of diseases was modelled upon Hippocrates, whom he much admired, but as befits one writing six hundred years later, he was rather more precise and academic. He also plagiarised the works of Rufus of Ephesus, although no great believer in the latter's concept of metastatic gout.

It was Aretaeus who first suggested that the cause of gout might lie in the presence in the blood of a specific "peccant humour" (toxic substance) rather than in a mere local plethora of one or more of the four humours constituting the normal body. It was not until Garrod's discovery, seventeen hundred years later, that this peccant humour consisted of uric acid, that Aretaeus' hypothesis became academically justified. It is generally agreed that he was one of the most talented and critical physicians of antiquity. His two great treatises, which he wrote for the Emperor Vespasian, still survive: *On the Causes of Acute and Chronic Diseases* and *On Their Treatment.* Although it sometimes seems in reading his works that, like Hippocrates and Soranus, he also recognised variants of the species "arthritis," he did not differentiate their treatment. His therapy, although traditional, was always reasonable and appears to have been based upon rational indications.

Aretaeus advocated hellebore as the sovereign remedy, "yet only in the first attacks of the affliction. If it has subsisted for a long time already and also if it appears to have been transmitted from the patient's forefathers, the disease sticks to him until death, and purgation or internal treatment is of no avail." Aretaeus appears to have thought, however, that hellebore might have some property more specific for gout than its mere purgative effect. He pointed out in discussion that it was not the most powerful purgative or emetic available, "for of the former, cholera can equal this; and of the violence of the vomiting, this seasickness can excell; but from a quality of no mean description it [hellebore] will restore the patient to health even with small purging and little retching." This may well be true since, as mentioned later, hellebore is related to colchicum. For chronic sufferers he thought strong internal medication inadvisable, but counter-irritation he believed might often be helpful.

Evidently he also recognised that the relatively non-vascular, deep tissues are not sensitive to the pain of incision. His words are worth quoting:

> The first affected [in gout] are the ligaments of the joints, such as have their origin in the bones. Now there is a great wonder in regard to these; there is not the slightest pain in them should you cut or squeeze them; but if they become spontaneously painful, as in the gout, no other pain is more severe than this, not iron screws, nor cords, not the wound of a dagger, nor burning fire, for all these may be had recourse to as cures for the still greater pains. And if one cut them whilst they are painful the smaller pain of the incision is obscured by the greater; and if it prevail, they experience pleasure in forgetting their former sufferings . . . in a word, any part which is very compact is insensible to touch or to a wound. For pain consists of an irritation, but what is compact cannot be inflamed, and hence is not sensible to pain; but a spongy tissue is very sensitive.

He noted as a prognostic fact that "in many cases the gout has passed into dropsy, and sometimes into asthma; and from this succession there is no escape but death." As further evidence of his clinical descriptive ability his account of the first onset of gout may be quoted and com-

pared with the more famous later description of Sydenham:

> The joints begin to be affected in this way; pain seizes the
> great toe, then the forepart of the heel on which we rest;
> next it comes into the arch of the foot, but the ankle-joint
> swells last of all. All sufferers at first wish to blame the
> wrong cause—some friction of a new shoe, others a long
> walk, others an accident, or being trodden upon . . . but
> the true cause is seldom believed by the patient when he
> hears it from the physician. On this account the disease
> often progresses to an incurable stage because at the com-
> mencement the physician is not consulted, whilst the dis-
> ease is feeble and can be brought under control. When it
> has acquired strength with time all treatment is useless.

He pointed out that in the "hot species" of arthritis,
by which he may have meant gout, local refrigeration is
more helpful than warmth, and advocated cold sea-water
baths followed by inunction of the joint with oil, or a
poultice of cucumber, lemon peel, plantain leaves, and
rose petals, wrapped in the unscoured wool of a sheep, to
which a little rose oil or wine was added periodically. For
excessive pain moistened cinquefoil and horehound leaves
might be added. He ended his chapter on medicines with
the sage words: "The medicines for this disease are in-
numerable; for the calamity and the pain thereof renders
the patients themselves very expert druggists."

After the fall of Rome at the close of the fourth century
A.D., Byzantium, later called Constantinople and now
Istanbul, became the centre of the Empire. Although
Galenism flourished in its new soil the Byzantine physi-
cians showed but little evidence of new thought in the
realm of gout. Many new and exotic remedies from the
East were introduced, but these were mostly of no value.
Aetius of Amida (fourth century), the first Christian
medical writer, who combined the posts of Lord High

Chamberlain and Court Physician to the Emperor Jus-
tinian, mentioned the virtue of magnets (lodestones) for
the relief of pain of gout in hands or feet if they be
strapped to them. He also decreed a regimen, different
for every month of the year, which would last for two
years. This was quoted with modified approval by the
eighteenth-century medical historian, Dr. John Freind.

Quackery was rife and many of the more absurd and
disgusting forms of treatment which found their way
later into Mediaeval Europe owed their origin to this
source and not to academic medicine as is often believed.
The one event of real importance which occurred at this
time was the introduction by Alexander of Tralles of
colchicum (hermodactyl) as a specific treatment for gout.
This fascinating story is considered more fully in the
next chapter.

Paul of Aegina (A.D. 625–690), the last of the great
Greek physicians of Byzantium, was responsible about
this time for codifying, and to some extent clarifying, the
heritage of Greek medicine and more particularly surgery. He thought that in addition to the basic humoral
abnormality envisaged by Hippocrates in gout, there must
also be some congenital weakness or mechanical inferi-
ority of any joint which would attract and fix the gouty
humour, and that when the "morbid principle" was in
great excess it would ooze through the coverings of the
joint and crystallize out as tophi. He was one of the first
to record his belief that attacks are precipitated as the
result of sorrow, anxiety, or other passions of the mind.
Of hermodactyl he agreed that "sodden by itself it do
purge the belly, and helpeth morbus articularis, which
is the sickness of the joyntes; as the goute, the sciatice,
and the paynes in the joyntes of the handes called cyagra."
It appears that he used an infusion of the whole plant,

unlike Alexander of Tralles who employed only the corm.

In the eighth century, medicine passed into the keeping of the Moslem Empire, and the teachings of Galen once again survived triumphantly this new implantation. The great physicians of the Caliphate—Mesue (d. 857), Rhazes (d. 923–924), and Avicenna (980–1037), the "Prince of Physicians"—applied the new botanical knowledge which was seeping in from India, Persia, and possibly even China, to the materia medica, but, for gout, colchicum remained the standard remedy, unchanged.

CHAPTER III

The Story of Colchicum

After the fall of Rome, Constantinople became the capital of the arts and sciences of the ancient world. Not much of value was added to medicine by the Byzantine physicians except for the introduction of some empirical Eastern remedies, and it is here that the history of the use of hermodactyl, or colchicum, for the treatment of gout begins. It is true that it had been used occasionally by the ancient Greeks as a powerful purgative, but there is very little evidence that they suspected that it might possess any more specific properties for the treatment of this disease. Moreover, Dioscorides had written of it as a deadly poison with which unhappy slaves would often end their lives. It is not until we meet those surviving portions of the voluminous writings of the Byzantine Christian physician, Alexander of Tralles, whose brother designed the great church of Sancta Sophia, that we can read of its selective and specific properties for the first time. He recognised, however, that it was not helpful in every case of "arthritis," and wisely postulated that there might be many varieties of the arthritic disease and thus many types of remedies might be needed.

Hermodactyl appears to have been extracted by him from the corm of a large species of colchicum (*C. variegatum*), similar to but not identical with the more effective *Colchicum autumnale*. This is a crocus-like plant named from the fact that it was originally imported from Colchis in Asia Minor; although it also grows to some extent along all the eastern shores of the Mediterranean, as do many other varieties with which no doubt it was often confused. It is of the genus *Melanthaceae* and so is a cousin of the white hellebore which was recommended by Hippocrates and his followers as a "sovereign purge" for the gout.

Alexander of Tralles gives the following formula for the preparation of hermodactyl: "Of the dried corm take four scruples, of scammony two scruples, and suspend in warm water. Then give this to the patient, who must have been well prepared for three days by the proper regimen." He described graphically the immense relief from pain and swelling of the joints experienced by many of his patients within a very short time.

Another Christian physician of Byzantium, Aetius, also advocated its use, but was aware of its side effects, as he says:

> It rapidly calms the pain, generally within two days, and permits the sufferer to resume his usual occupation—but caution must be observed that this relief be not unduly expedited. Some in the paroxysms of arthritic disease have recourse to hermodactyl in great doses, but it is to be remarked that hermodactyl is bad for the stomach, producing nausea and anorexia, and ought therefore only to be used in the case of those who are pressed for time by urgent affairs of business, for it does remove the disease quickly, after two days at most, so that they are enabled to resume. For this reason some do call it *anima articulorum*—the soul of the joints.

Because of the gastric irritation which hermodactyl produced as a side effect, Aetius was accustomed to prescribe certain aromatic spices with it which he thought would mitigate this, as did Paul of Aegina and no doubt many of the later physicians.

Colchicum was closely studied by the botanical physicians of the subsequent Moslem Empire, perhaps partly on account of its reputed aphrodisiac property, and its use was continued in gout throughout the period of the Caliphates until the eighteenth century. Caelius Aurelianus, the distinguished Roman physician who practised during the fifth century in Carthage—for a short period prior to its conquest by the Moslems the centre of the western portion of the Empire—had made colchicum well known throughout southern Europe through his writings, so that when the Moslems invaded from North Africa and conquered portions of Spain and Italy, and with the establishment of the first European medical school at Salerno near Naples, the virtue of colchicum for the treatment of gout was already known and was taught in the school. The famous Salernitan *Regimen* says of the *Bulbus rusticus,* the Latin name for colchicum: "We know that it helpeth the arthritic gout and the pellagra."

The first pharmacopoeia, which dates from this period, the *Antidotary* of Nicholas, contains hermodactyl as a constituent of *Pil. arthritica,* of which there were two varieties, one for use during the summer and the other for winter use. Its sinister reputation as a potent poison, which had been much written up by Dioscorides and Pliny, however, appealed greatly to the mediaeval mind, and this may have limited its popularity for more legitimate purposes. The formidable Abbess Hildegard of Bingen, whose influence spread all through Germany, actually forbade its use, saying that "it is a deadly poison and not a health-giving drug." So in the wild polypharmacy which became current practice throughout the Middle Ages in Europe, the use of colchicum as an ingredient in purgative and other mixtures was largely dropped. A further factor may have been the difficulty of obtaining and identifying the genuine corms, and in getting them properly dried and prepared. Nicholas thought it essential, if their potency was to be retained, that corms must be gathered in the spring and dried for a short time in the sun, after which they were to be hung in the dark at an even temperature and their coverings not damaged in any way for at least six months. Thus knowledge of its specific virtue became lost, except perhaps to certain peripatetic herbalists and "empirics" who continued to enjoy considerable success amongst the gouty upper class. Such was Gilbert Anglicus, who in the thirteenth century named the preparation of colchicum which he used "Cothopcie Alexanderine" in honour of its original discoverer.

Scudamore quotes the last reference to the specific use of colchicum in mediaeval Europe as contained in a prescription written for the Byzantine Emperor Michael Paleologus VIII in 1282 by his private physician: a small safe quantity of hermodactyl was combined with a very adequate dose of aloes and some mucilage. This prescription was accompanied with some sensible dietetic advice and the laconic message "This will cure you provided we have the assistance of Heaven, the intercession of the Blessed Virgin Mother, and the help of God."

Although for these various reasons colchicum practically ceased to be used by the physicians during the Middle Ages, it remained known to the botanists and herbalists, and so came once more to the notice of the academic physicians in the sixteenth century. These men were intolerant of anything of which the Moslems had approved, and so dismissed it as merely an old-fashioned purgative whose action was too violent to render it of practical use. The physician William Turner, who is often known as the father of scientific botany in England, wrote in his *Herbal* (1548): "Colchicum is abused [mistaken] by some poticaries for Hermodactylus. Colchicum hath leaves and

seedes in Sommer, and flowres lyke saffron aboute Michel-
masse. It maye be called in Englysshe Wylde Saffron."
But he counselled against its use. William Bullein, a
learned physician of Elizabethan England, wrote in his
Boke of Compoundes (1579):

> Hermodactyl be of ii kindes, the first is colchicum wyld
> bulbus, or greate wyld saffron having greate rounde leaves
> within the grounde, like to onions . . . the seconde is lyke
> a lyllie with tender leaves, white flowers, bitter seede, one
> large roote and the bigness of a finger. Both these Hermo-
> dactyles be called Mercuryes fingers, as sayeth Galen, de-
> scribing the same as aforesaid with the same vertues. It is
> well that it be not used.

In fact there were many other kinds of corm which passed
as the genuine colchicum at that time, even amongst the
botanists.

The apothecary, John Gerard, also described it (1597)
and mentioned that "It can be very hurtfull to the stomach." He added that it may prove effective for joint pains,
however, "when mixed with white of eggs, barley meal
and crumbs of bread and applied plaister-wise"; and
sometimes even if the corm be merely carried round in
the pocket or worn round the neck. These alternative
methods of use would seem to be aiming to eliminate the
toxic oral effects which physicians, whose materia medica
was still based on Dioscorides, so much feared. According
to Leonhart Fuchs (1542), always a practical man, it had
the further advantage, when used in this latter way, that
it killed the fleas on the wearer's person.

It remained traditional to treat gout by purgation, however, and small doses of native-grown colchicum were
sometimes still introduced as a constituent of such mixtures. Therefore, no doubt, a sufferer might occasionally

receive a draught which contained colchicum and so would be relieved of his pain; and thus the reputation of traditional cathartic therapy was perpetuated. Hermodactyl appears amongst the simples listed in the first edition of the *Pharmacopoeia Londinensis* (1618), but was dropped subsequently until the edition of 1788. This was because the great Sydenham decreed, out of his personal experience, that all purgative treatments were bad because they "bring on what they were meant to keep off." As the result of this advice from such an influential source, purgative prescriptions for the gout all over Europe were scrapped, and hence the use of colchicum again effectively ceased.

It remained in oblivion until its rediscovery in 1763 by Professor Baron Von Stoerk, a pupil of Boerhaave, who was head of the Medical Clinic in Vienna and physician to the Empress Maria Theresa. According to Delpeuch, he was the first to establish with certainty that it was possible to ingest small quantities of this deadly poison regularly for a time without risking sudden death, and that the patient might even benefit from such temerity. He advocated its virtues principally in the treatment of dropsy, however, so it was not until the early part of the nineteenth century that its specific value in the treatment of gout became universally acknowledged.

This came about chiefly as the result of the great success which was enjoyed throughout Europe by Husson's patent medicine, L'Eau d'Husson. He had put this on sale from about 1780 onwards, but refused to divulge its contents. As the result of opposition aroused in the medical profession, and the fact that Husson advertised it extensively as a specific for most of the ills to which the flesh is heir, the police prohibited its sale for a short time.

Its beneficial effects upon the gout were so undoubted, however, that the ban had to be lifted.

The first English sufferer to experience this benefit was a Mr. John Crawfurd, whose doctor, Dr. Edwin Godden Jones, introduced the remedy into England in 1808 after considerable trial in his practice. He then wrote a small book entitled *An Account of the Remarkable Effects of the Eau Médicinale d'Husson in the Gout* (1810), which he dedicated to the Prince Regent's physician, Sir Walter Farquhar, who refused, however, to use the secret formula on his royal patient.

In 1814 Dr. James Want discovered that the basic ingredient was colchicum, and he published this finding in *The Medical and Physical Journal* together with a suggested formula for preparing a tincture. Monsieur Husson, however, had found a better way of standardising and preserving this substance, and shortly afterwards an agency for its sale was opened at the corner of St. James's Street, London. A few bottles had been brought from France in 1810 by a friend for Sir Joseph Banks, the venerable President of the Royal Society, who also reported considerable success in his own case, thereby surprising his somewhat orthodox physician, Sir Everard Home, who at once started to investigate its properties. Home was soon extolling the virtues of his personal recipe according to which he maintained two pounds of the macerated roots at a gentle heat in twenty-four ounces of sherry wine for six days before bottling it. In 1817 King George IV is reported to have announced to his personal physicians, Sir Henry Halford and Sir John Knighton: "Gentlemen, I have taken your half-measures long enough to please you. . . . From now on I shall take colchicum to please myself." At this time he was ingesting

1,200 drops of laudanum daily without relief of pain. The colchicum, however, helped him greatly. With the aid of colchicum, advised by the King, the gouty Bourbon Prince Louis was enabled to recover his health sufficiently to be restored from a somewhat sedentary existence in Richmond to the throne of France in 1815 as Louis XVIII.

These successes initiated a further spate of proprietary specifics of which one of the most controversial was "Moore's Wine of White Hellebore and Laudanum." Of this Scudamore reported in positive fashion: "I am well persuaded that in any form or combination it should be entirely deprecated as a remedy for the gout." "Dr. Wilson's Specific" also enjoyed considerable notoriety. Its discoverer presented some bottles to the Prince Regent, which Sir Henry Halford sternly forbade him to take.

Within a year or two the use of colchicum had once more become general throughout Europe for the treatment of this common affliction. In her *Memoir of the Reverend Sydney Smith* (1855) his daughter, Lady Holland, relates of this celebrated wit that on one occasion "on observing some of his autumn crocus in flower, he stopped; 'There,' he said, 'who would guess the virtue of that little plant? But I find the power of *colchicum* so great that if I feel a little gout coming on, I go into the garden and hold out my toe to that plant, and it gets well immediately. I never do more without orders from my physician.' " It is believed by Talbott that the bulbs were introduced into the United States by Benjamin Franklin who had successfully used colchicum for his gout whilst he was serving as ambassador in Paris.

Most of the great physicians of the nineteenth century, led by Sir Charles Scudamore, adopted the use of colchi-

cum enthusiastically and had their favourite methods
of preparation. Trousseau, the celebrated French consultant, alone held out against it, thinking that the side
effects of the unstandardised preparations then available
were too serious to justify its use. Gairdner also was not
alone in suggesting that although colchicum was undoubtedly useful in acute gout, it tended to aggravate the
underlying disease and, he believed, also increased the
frequency of the attacks. With the advance in chemical
techniques, however, these difficulties were overcome, and
in 1820 its active principle, the alkaloid colchicine, was
discovered by Pellétier and Caventou and produced in
crystalline form by Houdé in 1884. This soon replaced
the time-honoured tinctures, extracts, and other Galeni-
cal preparations of colchicum, as it was stable, reliable,
and easy to take in exact dosage, and its effective and
rapid control of pain in acute gout remained unrivalled.
Its method of action remains unknown, even today.

This is a strange page in medical history. Colchicum
was well studied, and had been known as an effective
remedy for certain painful and common affections of the
joints for a thousand years in the East. For a further three
centuries this knowledge was available and known to
some in the West. Then came the Renaissance and the
dominance of scholars who, with all this written and
practical evidence before them, chose to see none of it—
their learning seemed like a bandage round their eyes.
The use of colchicum, abandoned in this way by the
medical profession, was maintained throughout Europe
on a small scale by certain quacks and empirics until
eventually one of these produced a product which proved
so dramatically successful that it aroused the interest of
all Europe. It was to the discovery that the active princi-

ple of this Eau d'Husson consisted in colchicum, far more than to the poorly conducted and reported experiments of Von Stoerk, to whom credit is generally ascribed. Thus the re-introduction into medicine of one of the few natural specifics known to man took place.

CHAPTER IV

Gout at the Time of the Renaissance

The European Renaissance of learning did not mark any progress in man's understanding of gout. This seems curious as the spirit of the times was making for a climate of opinion highly critical of the theories and achievements of preceding centuries. In this sense medicine was comparatively immune, however, as progress in this art was judged to lie finally in the recovery of the pure texts of the ancient Greek masters, and the replacement by these of the works of the Moslems and mediaeval scholastics. The humoral hypothesis was not to come under fire for a further two centuries, although a gradual swing can be detected from the "pure" humoralism of Galen to a somewhat less doctrinaire conception which could be tailored to meet special circumstances. Thus it began to be thought that gout might not be owing only to an alteration in the proportion or nature of the humours, but might be caused by some chemical change in the blood, or even the production in the body of some unrelated toxic substance. Men became interested accordingly in the possible nature of such a substance and the site of its formation and storage in the body.

In England gout had been a well-recognised clinical entity, certainly since the thirteenth century. This may have been connected with the almost exclusively meat-eating habits of the nobility and upper classes. Vegetables were considered to be "food only for cottagers who can afford none other" and for members of the cloistered monastic orders who consumed them as evidence of the austerity of their regime. Fresh fruit also was seldom eaten by the educated, because on the infallible authority of "Pope Galen" it does engender the windy melancholy. The size of meals was enormous, and these were well washed down with the heavy, sweet wines of the Mediterranean coast.

The only seed of progress in the study of gout which seems to emerge from the literature from this time onwards may be discerned in the first English textbook of medicine, the *Rosa Anglica*, written in 1280 by John of Gaddesden, physician to King Henry V of England. In this he mentioned his personal observation that heredity in gout seemed to come more importantly through the mother's side of the family and might often skip a generation. He mentioned also that in his practice he kept two prescriptions of a purgative nature for the treatment of his patients: one for the rich and another for the poorer. It would not seem though that the latter class had firm grounds for any complaint regarding this undemocratic approach to their gout. The poor man's draught, it is true, did not contain electuary of pearls or the very special addition designed to strengthen their affected joints once the attack had passed, which was a powder of burnt human bone; but they got their purge.

Gout affected the Tudor dynasty from the outset, for the first of the Tudor Kings, Henry VII, was forced to postpone his marriage to the Princess Elizabeth, whereby the titles of York and Lancaster became finally united, on account of an attack of this disease, which we learn trailed him during the course of his reign. A little later the first specialist rheumatologist on record appears, one John Gilbert, who was licensed by King Henry VIII "to cure the goute, the crampe and all sore eyes." We have no knowledge, however, of his therapeutic methods. One of Henry's medical advisers, the priest-physician Andrew Boorde (1490–1549), wrote on the gout in his *Breviary of Healthe* (1542), and his views can be taken as expression of educated medical opinion in England, which at that time was still in the phase of mediaeval humoralism but was pleasantly tempered with empiricism and Anglo-Saxon folk-lore. Boorde tells us that the many causes of gout included the corruption of the humours by faulty diet or bad air and surroundings, an hereditary taint, and a native or adventitious weakness of the joints. Thomas Linacre, the foremost humanist physician of his time, himself appears to have subscribed to a magical viewpoint by sending in one year no less than twenty finger-rings, which had been blessed by the King, to some of his distinguished contemporaries abroad as cures for the rheumatism and the gout.

Treatment

Treatment was theoretically simple and consisted, Boorde said, in "opposing thereto those remedies contrary in quality and quantity to these causes." This also meant the elimination of the peccant humours by all possible means; prophylactic bleedings in spring and autumn, as Galen had advocated, together with a moderate dietary regime; and during attacks appropriate external remedies.

Boorde's more eclectic suggestions included the wearing of stockings (gaiters?) made of dog-skin, an idea which he may have got from the works of Soranus of Ephesus, who had suggested that gouty feet should be anointed with the fat of a seal and then encased in slippers made of its skin. Boorde also suggested the daily application to the painful joints of baked fermentations of ox dung wrapped in a cabbage leaf; and internally, fearsome scammony purges followed next day with large quantities of treacle to repair the damage and to "weaken the virulency of the gouty malignancy." This last treatment had also been advocated by Galen "to waste and weaken the thin virulent humour and dry it up." Boorde strongly recommended a watery infusion of the bark of the ash (*Fraxinus excelsior*), which became a favourite recipe all over Europe for gout and also for scurvy and fevers, as well as "for inflammations of the eyes, and to colour the hair black," until the introduction of the Peruvian bark (*Cinchona*) in the next century. The use of infusion of the leaves for some of these purposes still survives in parts of Southern England. Culpeper later thought the leaves of the dwarf elm tree more efficacious, and facetiously exhorted the sufferer "to drink it, being boiled in white wine; to drink the decoction I mean, not the Elm tree."

Boorde thought that diuresis was important and should be encouraged by the use of the roots of sorrel, parsley, and other herbs boiled in broth. We must record the warning issued by his contemporary author, Sir Thomas Elyot, however, who said that "Radysh rootes breaketh wind and doth provoke a man to make water, but they be verye evyl for them the wych hath the goute."

Throughout the later Middle Ages we find curious and often disgusting forms of treatment advocated by well-known practitioners. These may perhaps have been effective from their psychological impact, and the fact that they cannot have been easy to prepare. For instance, Lorenz Fries, a writer of popular medical works, in his *Spiegel der Artzny* (1518) advocated the following: "Roast a fat old goose and stuff with chopped kittens, lard, incense, wax and flour of rye. This must all be eaten, and the drippings applied to the painful joints. . . . It then withdraws the pains in the joints." Again, "the sodden flesh of a weasel or a cat, tied over a rheumatic joint, allays the pain," as does the fat of a fox well rubbed in. A "warm and bleeding pigeon" applied to the soles of the feet was also well thought of.

Singer believed gout to have been a very common disease amongst primitive peoples everywhere, and cites the leech-books of the Anglo-Saxons, who named it the "Fot-Adl." Spenser, in his *Faerie Queene* (1590) introduced a simple English peasant: "And eke in foote and hande a grievous goute tormented him full sore." Recent surveys have shown that it is still very common amongst the Maoris of New Zealand.

Examples of Saxon folk medicine are recorded in Frazer's *Golden Bough*. Sometimes the sufferer would recite a prayer or spell whilst tying a knot in the bough of a willow bush. For so long as he then kept away from this bush the gout would stay away from him. In magic all knots are symbolic of obstruction, and so of delaying power over a disease which might otherwise become chronic.

Nail parings and hair still have a high sympathetic magic value amongst all primitive peoples, and it was usual to place a portion of nail, together with some hairs cut from the lower part of the affected leg, into a hole in an oak tree trunk and fasten them in with cow dung. If during the next three months the sufferer remained free of attacks, then the disease would be transferred to the tree and he would suffer no more.

The unconventional views of the angry young rebel doctor, Paracelsus, have already been referred to. He made no practical advance in the therapy of gout but was the first to suggest the possibility of a chemical as opposed to a humoral causation for this disease in his tract, *De Morbis Tartareis* (1531). He believed that a tartarous material, which the body could neither digest nor excrete, became deposited in certain regions of the body. These sites included the teeth, where these deposits were the cause of toothache, the kidneys and bladder as calculi, and in and around the joints, causing gout. He thought that there might be some local factor such as the water supply, which influenced this chemical process, as he noted that in Switzerland "the most healthy land, superior to Germany, Italy and France, nay all Western and Eastern Europe, there is no gout, no colic, no rheumatisms and no stone." His teaching was carried on by Jean-Baptiste van Helmont, whose views, however, became even more mystical and incomprehensible to his colleagues, who accordingly lost interest.

Perhaps the most sophisticated contemporary discussion of gout is to be found in the section entitled "Of the disease of the joints commonly called the gout," in *The Most Excellent Workes of Master Ambrose Parey* (1634). This is a translation by the apothecary, Thomas Johnson, who also edited the second edition of the famous *Herball* of John Gerard, Lord Burghley's herbarist, and who was killed fighting gallantly for King Charles I in the siege of Basing House.

Ambroise Paré, the great French surgeon (1510–1590), wrote eloquently, being like Sydenham, a severe sufferer himself. He described his own case in Book XVIII of his *Workes* and declared: "The paines of the goute are rightly accounted amongst the most grievous and acute; so that through the vehemency of the agony many are almost mad, and wish themselves dead." He noted that the natural duration of an acute attack was forty days, although those who had developed tophi were scarcely ever free. He observed a stricter periodicity in the attacks of those who suffered with the inherited type of disease; and in some others a purely individual rhythm.

Paré's views on the origins of the disease were in the Galenic tradition. He pointed out, however, that it was the toxic virulence of the peccant matter distilled from the humours and not the quantity that was important, "as it causeth extreme paines not by abundance, because it happens to many who have no signe of swelling in the jointes." Of the mysterious nature of this matter he declared: "It is not of a more known nature than that which causeth the plague or the *Lues veneria*." He believed that in most cases the affected joint must previously have been weakened, either by nature or by accident.

As a "proof" that the major cause of gout lay in over-indulgence Paré remarked: "There have been, as I know, not a few rich and riotous persons, who having spent their estates, have therewith changed their health together with their fortune and their diet, and so have been wholly freed from the goute." Discussing dietetic regimes he advocated the use of chicken, but made the interesting point that "capon and suchlike birds are not good, being themselves subject to goute in their feet." It is mentioned elsewhere that hawks, which were much used at this time for sporting purposes, were also believed, like their masters, to be subject to this complaint.

Paré believed in a very vigorous all-out attack upon "the causative phlegmatic and serous humours" at an early age. This involved frequent copious bloodletting, vomits, sweating, diuresis, and purging; and it is interesting to note that one of the purges he recommended was hermodactyl pills.

He considered a permanent regime of temperance to be essential; indeed, he said: "Such gouty persons as remain intemperate and given to gluttony and venerie (especially the old) may hope for no health by the use of medicines." He also added that: "Neither can one and a like remedy be useful in every goute."

He warned against the use of narcotics except in extreme cases, and was cautious in the use of all external remedies with the exception of cauterisation and the use of setons. He emphasised that these must be applied only to the outer side of the knees and legs, however, to avoid subsequent difficulty in horseback riding should these wounds not heal readily. He also advised gouty subjects not to drink much, as he thought that fluid would cool the stomach and so arrest active metabolism, thus leaving "crudities" which could not be excreted and so would collect in the blood-stream. In later life he became less confident in his therapeutic potential, and referred to gout as the "Opprobrium Medicorum."

Some Notable Sufferers

The great Renaissance Italian family of Medici serves to illustrate the association between outstanding ability and the gouty diathesis which has been remarked by many observers throughout the ages. Cosimo de' Medici (1389–1464) was the son of the gouty Giovanni di Bicci de' Medici. Of Cosimo we learn that "he grew old very rapidly as he suffered very severely from the gout, and in his later years became very infirm, which caused him to leave the affairs of the state largely to others." Nonetheless, such was the honour and respect in which he was held that by public decree the title of "Father of his people" was conferred upon him posthumously; and by order of the Republic the honourable inscription: *Cosimus Medices hic situs est decreto publico Pater Patriae* was written upon his grave.

Cosimo had two sons of whom "Piero il Gottoso" (Peter

the Gouty, 1416–1469) succeeded him at the age of forty-eight as ruler of Florence. He had suffered with attacks of acute gout from boyhood, hence his soubriquet. This affliction handicapped him greatly through life as for long periods he became unable to take part in public affairs. Piero became very crippled towards the end of his life and eventually his disablement was so complete that he was able to use only his tongue. He died at the age of fifty-three, being succeeded by his young son, Lorenzo the Magnificent (1449–1492), who although he inherited the family gout, was less severely afflicted than his father and grandfather, and lived to enhance Medicean patronage of the arts, of which Michelangelo, another sufferer, was the chief glory.

The Holy Roman Emperor Charles V (1500–1558) suffered his first acute attack of gout at the age of twenty-eight, and was almost continuously physically incapacitated by 1550. Each attack made an incisive impact upon his memory as he recorded the time and place of each in his memoirs. In spite of the physical restraint which his increasing incapacity laid upon his martial, diplomatic, and other ambitions, Charles is said to have been consistently unable to control the gluttonous and abnormal appetite which fostered his disease. So in spite of the conscientious efforts of his regular medical advisers, who included the great Vesalius, he was ever ready to give ear to the suggestions of the newest quack who would promise him a quick recovery without dietetic restriction.

His vast possessions, both in Europe and in the New World, and the continual threat of Turkish invasion, entailed enormous and inescapable responsibilities and decisions which could only rest with the ruler personally. In such circumstances the state of his health must ultimately have influenced the fate of these territories greatly.

His increasingly recurrent bouts of gout and the resultant
incapacity were observed by his contemporaries to affect
Imperial affairs in many spheres, often by preventing
prompt decisions and leaving much important business
unfinished for long periods of time. So it was, for example, in the course of war with France, that in 1552
plans to lay siege to Metz, the key to Lorraine and Champagne, had to be postponed for the sake of the emperor's
gout. The long delay permitted the French to strengthen
the fortress so that what would have been a relatively
easy victory of great significance for the Imperialists had
to be foregone with consequent extension of the war and
its problems. Such enforced inefficiency and its resulting
frustrations in the greatest ruler in Christendom tended
to emphasise a preëxistent depressive state which led him
finally to his unprecedented act of abdicating the Imperial
throne in 1556; and two years later he died miserably
"sicke and frustrated of the goute before the High Altar
of his chapel in the Escorial."
    The newly fashionable remedy for gout and many
diseases at this time was a decoction of the guaiac wood,
or *Lignum vitae,* which had recently been introduced
from the New World and for which the millionaire bank-
ing family of Fugger in Augsburg had the monopoly of
import into Europe. An even newer alternative was what
was known as the China root, probably the diuretic extract of the dried rhizome known later as *Smilax china,*
brought back by the Portuguese navigators, for which
similar virtues were claimed. Vesalius wrote a treatise on
this wonder-drug in 1546. In either case the patient was
put to bed in an heated room on a low diet, and the decoction was administered at frequent intervals until the
attack subsided, which would often take a month or more.
The Emperor was naturally subjected to each of these

"specifics"; he preferred the China root, however, as less dietetic restriction was thought necessary with its use. Both remedies shortly died a natural death.

Charles's son, Philip II of Spain, who married Mary Tudor, Queen of England, suffered his first inherited twinges of gout six years after his accession to the throne of the Spanish Empire. And ten years later the disease had become chronic, entailing constant pain and much immobility. A chronicler comments on his passive appearance at this time: "His cane-coloured hair and beard, and the tepid blue moleskin-soft eyes that not even cruelty could now fan into flame." He was careful in his fanatical piety not to have his disease treated, as he regarded the affliction as God's rebuke to a servant who was not being sufficiently diligent in the holy work of exterminating heretics. He therefore devoted himself thereafter more fully to organising what P. M. Dale called the unspeakable cruelties inflicted by a man, not basically inhumane, upon the hapless victims of the Spanish Inquisition. It was from this time of its ruler's disease-determined shift of interest from the affairs of state that the decline of Spain as a great power was accelerated.

It is recorded that no word of complaint as to his lot was ever heard throughout his long life. By the age of sixty-five Philip had become completely bedridden, unable to dress or feed himself, and from now onwards his surgeons were allowed to treat him, and they took full advantage. They bled him copiously and daily; they inserted setons around his joints which led to septic open sinuses and bed-sores, and the stench of his bedchamber was said to be more than his attendants could bear. He died, probably of toxaemia, on 12 September 1598.

Northern Europe also had its important sufferers. The reformers, Martin Luther and John Calvin, were both victims of gout, and this affliction may well also have played its part in exacerbating the bitterness and cruelties of the Reformation in their lands.

A further, equally influential victim at this time was William Cecil, First Baron Burghley (1520–1598), Lord Treasurer of England, whose medical history is of considerable interest. The gout of a Prime Minister must in any time and in any important country attract the attention of the medical and lay public. This was particularly so at this formative period, the England of Elizabeth I, when the great Lord Burghley was leading her to the heights of world power. He was a considerable sufferer.

Burghley went up to St. John's College, Cambridge, then "the most famous place of education in England," when he was fifteen. There he met John Cheke, "whom men esteemed the profoundest Greek scholar of his time, whose widowed mother, to support her family had been driven to keep a small wine shop in the town." They became devoted friends and this took Burghley there, according to the records, "more frequently than was prudent." He was shortly removed from Cambridge without a degree, but later married Mary Cheke, the daughter of the house.

He then entered Gray's Inn and soon came to the notice of the King, and seemed assured of a brilliant career. Stamford elected him Member of Parliament in 1547, and he was made a Secretary of State in 1550. From then, until his death, he "continued to occupy a position in the affairs of the nation such as no other man in Europe below the rank of sovereign attained to."

At the age of thirty-three his first acute attack of gout necessitated a temporary retirement (1553), so when "Bloody Mary" Tudor succeeded as Queen he was out of office, and as she did not reinstate him he was powerless to oppose her marriage to Philip II of Spain. Her vigorous attempts to reverse the Reformation and the tragedy of the burning of the Smithfield martyrs, disgusted him. Parliament met in October, 1555, to consider, at her request, a measure for confiscating the estates of those Protestant gentry who had fled from her persecution, and Cecil succeeded in getting this bill thrown out and shortly afterwards got into secret touch with the Princess Elizabeth.

On her accession in 1558 as Queen, he was appointed Chief Secretary of State, of which the modern equivalent is Prime Minister, and owing to another sudden and prolonged attack of his gout she held her first audience in his house at Hatfield and assumed her government from there. His responsibility "stresses" at this time included lack of money, the constant plotting by the Pope and English Catholics, and the threat of invasion from France and Scotland, with all of which he successfully dealt.

When Elizabeth withdrew somewhat during the next year from routine business to amuse herself with Lord Robert Dudley, however, Burghley's health again began to suffer under the strain of constant labour, of mind and body. This showed as a succession of minor break-downs characterised by acute attacks of gout. As the result of one of these he signed the Treaty of Edinburgh whilst in great pain, so making some concessions regarding the possible succession to the English throne of Mary, Queen of Scots, that so much annoyed Elizabeth that he lost his influence with her almost completely for a time. This he only recovered when the prevailing unrest in the country became so great that she had to appoint a Commission of Inquiry of which he was the only acceptable chairman. The unexampled provocation which this one-man government endured during the next few years included daily risk of assassination until the Popish menace was ended with the final defeat of the Spanish Armada. It is evident that the resultant stresses produced frequent acute attacks, which must often have affected his outlook and perhaps his policy.

As his sufferings in this respect were well known it is not surprising that one of the most usual of the many gifts which were sent to him from all over the civilised world from admirers or candidates for the favour of the most powerful man in the kingdom, took the form of secret and often exotic prescriptions to cure these attacks. Amongst the *Lansdowne Manuscripts* in the British Museum there are letters to Lord Burghley from all parts of Europe, in English, Latin, French, and Italian, offering him nostrums of the most infallible kind.

The first of these is a letter from a Mr. Dyon, dated 24 January 1553, at which time Burghley was thirty-three years old, recommending him to pursue a certain course of diet and physic which is marked on the outside in Lord Burghley's handwriting *Recipe pro podagra*. There are other directions of a similar nature from the Lady Harington (1573), and an Italian letter concerning a special secret powder for the gout, dated the 12 December 1575. Four years later Dr. Henry Landwer sent him a prescription in Latin for medicated slippers to relieve his gout; whilst Dr. Hector Nones (or Nunez), one of the heads of the Spanish Jewish colony in London and a Fellow of the College of Physicians, bombarded him regularly with remedies selected from the works of Averroes, Joannes Anglicus, and Matthaeus de Gradibus. In 1583 another letter was received from one Nicholas Gybberd who pretended to have discovered an infallible cure in the form of an alchemical tincture of gold. The Earl of Shrewsbury also wrote heartily wishing that His Lordship "wolde make trial of my OYLE OF STAGS BLUD, for I am strongly persuaded of the rare and great vertu thereof. I know it to be a most safe thynge, yet some offence there is in the smell thereof."

The following letter was sent in 1592 by Henry Bossevyle, an alchemist living in Calais, offering for a fee of four or five hundred pounds and suitable preferment, to "furnish some infallible plaisters to cure the gout."

> My goode Lord—Touchinge the substance of the things that go to this cure the styll is used, and there are several waters and things spread upon a certayne beste skynne made leather. Concernynge the applyinge thereof, one water [solution] must bathe the place nere unto the payne, leaving a joynte between the place of payne and the place bathed, if conveniently it maye be. Then must a peece of the sayd lether be cutte convenient to make a plaister, which muste be well moystened in one of the sayde waters, and thereon severall other powerful things spredde, which plaister muste be layde upon the place bathed, there to remayne XII howers; and afterwards there must be freshe bathinge and plaisters.
>
> For the operacion thereof the paciente shall shortly fynde the humore stirred, blisters or pymples to rise where the plaister is layde, out of which shall yssue the badde humore, some of which blisters wyll drye up, and others wyll unely breake out so longe as any parte of the humore remaynethe.
>
> When all the badde humore is drawne out they will drye up and the paciente shall fynde hymself for the present cured, by havinge the use of his joynts as nymble as ever they were, and afterwardes shall feele no more payne of the gout. . . . I do affirme yt upon my faythe, that besides the laboure and charges of the things that go to the cure . . . yt hath coste me more fayre gold than I thinke was ever given in England for a medecyne. (*Lansdowne Manuscripts*, British Museum, no. 69, art. 60).

It seems, however, that Lord Burghley preferred his disease to this remedy, as no answer was sent.

From 1572, when he was created Lord High Treasurer of England, until his death, to write of his career, in the words of Froude, "is to write the history of England; for by him more than by any other single person was the history of England shaped." Can we doubt, therefore, that his increasingly frequent, lengthy, and painful attacks of gout influenced the history of his country and of Europe at that time and for many years afterwards? Some day further and more detailed evidence of this will be extracted from the State Papers where it undoubtedly exists.

To his son, Robert (1563?–1612), Earl of Salisbury and successor to several of his offices of state, Burghley also bequeathed his gout, from which indeed Robert died on 24 May 1612, on his return from a "cure" in Bath which had been ordered by Sir Theodore Mayerne, the Royal Physician. Burghley's eldest son, Thomas (1542–1622), Earl of Exeter, also suffered to some considerable extent, which led to his retirement from court life and confined him to his house at Wimbledon intermittently until his death.

To bring the story up to date, it is interesting to note that neither the present Lord Burghley (now Marquess of Exeter), nor his late father has suffered from gout, although there remains a familial tendency to degenerative joint disease.

In 1583 Dr. Philip Barrough, a Fellow of the College of Physicians, published his *Method of Phisicke*, which he dedicated to Lord Burghley. In the chapter entitled "Of the goute in the feet and the jointes," he discussed the causes of the disease and mentions, with a seemingly curious lack of tact, that "this disease is engendered of continued crudities and drunkeness, and of immoderate using of lechery."

Shakespeare's pithy comment upon the hopeless outlook for the chronic gouty sufferer of his time—whose only release was death—is expressed in *Cymbaline:*

> One that's sick o' the gout would rather
> Groan so in perplexity than be cured
> By th' one sure physician, Death.

In Tudor times gout was apparently not considered the prerogative solely of the human species, but also afflicted horses, capons, and falcons, which last were much used for sporting and "prestige" purposes. In Turberville's *Faulconrie* (1575) it is pointed out that "many times . . . a goute doth befall a hawke, which is none other thinge than a hard tumor and swelling full of corruption about the joyntes of a hawkes foote and stretchers." We are also informed that "olde nightingales kepte in a cage are subject to the gowte." The cure for this avian variety of the disease was to be found in the native herb named the Gout-wort, or *Herba Gerardi,* which is described in Gerard's *Herball.* He tells us that "the roots of this are to be well 'stamped' and laid upon the swelling. This will result in the assuagement of the malign humours, and so cure." Culpeper was even more explicit, saying: "The very bearing of it eases the pains of the gout in man and beast and defends him that bears it from the disease."

CHAPTER V

Gout in the Seventeenth Century

The story of gout during the seventeenth century is largely that of Thomas Sydenham (1624–1689), whom his countrymen named in admiration the English Hippocrates. His classic description of the disease, which was based upon his own sufferings, wherein he differentiated finally between gout and rheumatism, has never been surpassed. As to its treatment, although warning against the dangers of so-called gouty specifics, he suggested, with charming modesty, that since he had suffered from the unrelenting attentions of the disease for thirty-four years his observations on its cure might not carry very much weight.

His prohibition of the use of the violent purges usual at that time proved unfortunate for his fellow sufferers, as scammony and colocynth, together with a small dose of colchicum, formed the basis for most purgative prescriptions, and this resulted in the use of colchicum being banished throughout Europe for the next hundred and fifty years.

Whilst serving as a combatant officer in the rebel army of Cromwell, a fellow victim of the disease, at the age of thirty-seven, seven years after his first attack of gout, Sydenham developed haematuria from a renal calculus and was subsequently seldom out of pain. No doubt this helped to condition that rather sombre outlook on life which is reflected in his writings. Soon his work became interrupted almost annually for long periods by attacks, during which, as he wrote, he found himself "unable to indulge in any deep train of thought" for fear of their exacerbation.

His famous *Treatise on the Gout* (1683) was written at the request of Dr. Thomas Short, the historically-minded Master of Gonville and Caius College, who became the Regius Professor at Cambridge. In its preface he apologises for its brevity, saying that "my health prevents me from troubling the world much more with medical treatises . . . I am at a loss to know whether the stone or the gout be most severe." Soon after this he retired permanently to the country, for he had always complained that: "The town air is full of vapours, and is rendered still denser by the closeness of the buildings, especially in London, which is esteemed the largest City in the Universe." The population of London at that time was 670,000. His other intention was to "go to bed early, especially in the winter."

The therapeutic methods he advocated were simple, direct, and largely what we would call "expectant." They owed little to the works of his predecessors or contemporaries, which he pretended he had not even read. They comprised dietetic restriction, simple cooking, few drugs, and an ample, non-alcoholic fluid intake. Like Hippocrates Sydenham advocated for this last purpose a sort of barley water which he referred to as his "diet-drink." Advice of this nature was not usual at this period. An impartial observer of English habits, Bernardino Ramazzini of Padua, recorded in his *De Morbis Artificium* (English translation, 1746) that in England: "The people of distinction and opulence indulge themselves . . . eating the most rich and luscious fleshes in great quantity, and drink large amounts of generous wines. By this means Nature is rendered incapable of managing the large quantity of blood, and carrying off the secretions which ought to be made from it."

Sydenham also advocated a tranquil life devoid of excesses, preferably in the country, with regular horse-back exercise. He was greatly averse to the drastic purging and bleeding which were usual in his time to remove the "peccant humours" of gout, and confined himself to the use of a few herbal remedies. Opium was his favourite medicament during the acute attack, and he introduced a liquid tincture of laudanum which brought him early fame throughout the continent of Europe. He used the newly introduced Jesuits' bark (quinine) as a prophylactic between attacks. He advocated minimal interference with the acute attack as he considered that "this pain is the disagreeable remedy of Nature herself." Regarding the use of analgesic applications he was sceptical, saying of them: "To ease the pain in the gout I know of none (though I have tried abundance in myself and others) beside coolers and repellants which I have already shown to be unsafe . . . let them be used [by the patient] in the beginning of a fit and he will soon be convinced of their insignificancy."

Scudamore, commenting much later, remarked of Sydenham's system of treatment that "in view of his self-confessed suffering, the policy of leaving the cure of this disease largely in the hands of the nurse and the *vix medicatrix naturae* seems to have been discountenanced." Sydenham, however, was no nihilist, for he also wrote: "The radical cure of the gout is yet a secret; but after long consideration I cannot help thinking that a [specific] remedy will be found out hereafter."

Many of the descriptive portions of his *Treatise* remain worthy of reading today, and a small extract will be quoted. This work was originally intended by him to have been part of a larger work on the chronic diseases, "had my pains spared me somewhat . . . but too much study and business is pernicious for me . . . and hence I conceive it is that so few fools have had the gout." Since naturally he was a believer in the humoral hypothesis his therapeutic views are of less current interest; although we cannot but lend a sympathetic ear from the safety of the twentieth century to his pithy comment: "I scruple not to affirm from a long course of experience that most of those who are supposed to perish of the gout are rather destroyed by wrong management than by the disease itself." Bearing upon this aspect, however, we find John Graunt writing in his *Bills of Mortality* (1662), the forerunner of all statistical surveys of the public health: "There dies not above one of a thousand of the gout, although I believe that many die gouty." Graunt, an army officer with a pioneer interest in vital statistics, was later falsely accused of having started the Great Fire of London!

The first treatise to be written on the gout in English was that of Dr. Benjamin Welles, a Fellow of All Souls who retired to practise near Greenwich on account of his depressive neurosis. This work, *A Treatise of the Gout, or Joint Evil* (1669), is dedicated to "My Arthritic patients—who now walk stoutly supported by my Art, as much as by their own leggs." Only three copies seem to have survived, two in London and one at Yale, and it is only such rarity, as well as precedence, that permits it to be mentioned in conjunction with Sydenham's celebrated treatise which will now be considered.

The Treatise on the Gout

As Sydenham wrote:

> There is no doubt but that men will conclude either that the nature of the disease, which is my present subject, is incomprehensible, or that I who have been afflicted with it for these thirty-four years past am a person of very slender

abilities—insomuch as my observations concerning this distemper and the cure thereof fall short of their expectations. But notwithstanding this I will faithfully deliver my remarks concerning the difficulties and intricacies occurring in the history of the disease and the method of cure, leaving the illustration thereof to time, that discoverer of the truth.

He goes on to mention that the disease is commonest amongst elderly people living lives of luxury, particularly those who, having been athletic in youth, have entirely given up exercise. "The gout, however, does not only seize the gross and corpulent, but sometimes, though less frequently, attacks lean and slender persons . . . sometimes in the prime of life, when they have received the seeds of it from gouty parents, or have otherwise occasioned it by an over-early use of venery."

The *regular gout* generally seizes in the following manner: it comes on a sudden towards the close of January or the beginning of February, giving scarce any sign of its approach except that the patient has been afflicted for some weeks before with a bad digestion . . . and the day preceding [*sic*] the fit the appetite is sharp but preternatural. The patient goes to bed and sleeps quietly till about two in the morning, when he is awakened by a pain which usually seizes the great toe, but sometimes the heel, the calf of the leg or the ankle. The pain resembles that of a dislocated bone . . . and this is immediately succeeded by a chillness, shivering and a slight fever. The chillness and shivering abate in proportion as the pain increases, which is mild in the beginning but grows gradually more violent every hour, and comes to its height towards evening, adapting itself to the numerous bones of the tarsus and metatarsus, the ligaments whereof it affects; sometimes resembling a tension or laceration of those ligaments, sometimes the gnawing of a dog, and sometimes a weight and constriction of the parts affected, which become so exquisitely painful as not to endure the weight of the clothes nor the shaking of the room from a person's walking briskly therein. And hence the

night is not only passed in pain, but likewise with number-
less endeavours to ease the pain by continually changing the
situation of the body and part affected, which notwithstanding abates not till two or three in the morning; that
is till after twenty-four hours from the first approach of the
fit, when the patient is suddenly relieved. . . . And being
now in a breathing sweat he falls asleep, and upon waking
finds the pain much abated, and the part affected to be then
swollen; whereas before only a remarkable swelling of the
veins thereof appeared, as is usual in all gouty fits.

The next day, and perhaps two or three days afterwards,
if the gouty matter be copious, the part affected will be
somewhat pained, and the pain increases towards evening
and remits about the break of day. In a few days it seizes
the other foot in the same manner, and if the pain be
violent in this, and that which was first seized be quite easy,
the weakness of this soon vanishes and it becomes as strong
and healthy as if it had never been indisposed; nevertheless the gout affects the foot just seized as it did the former,
both in respect of the vehemence and duration of the pain;
and sometimes . . . it affects both at the same time with
equal violence.

He points out that an attack of gout is always comprised
of a number of these recurrences or exacerbations, and
will often last two months, although those who possess
"strong constitutions, and such as seldom have the gout"
may recover in fourteen days. In patients who suffer frequent attacks or who are debilitated from age or disease,
the attack may last until the end of the following summer,
when it usually disappears.

During the first fourteen days the urine is high coloured,
and after separation lets fall a kind of red gravelly sedi-
ment, and not above a third part of the liquids taken in is
voided by urine, and the body is generally costive during
this time. The fit is accompanied throughout with loss of
appetite, chillness of the whole body towards eventide, and
a heaviness and uneasiness even of those parts that are not

affected by the disease. When the fit is going off a violent itching seizes the foot, especially between the toes, whence the skin peels off, as if the patient had taken poison. The disease being over, the appetite and strength return sooner or later, according as the immediately preceding fit hath been more or less severe, and in consequence of this the following fit comes on in a shorter or longer space of time; for if the last fit proved very violent the next will not attack the patient till the same season of the year returns again.

In this manner does the *regular gout,* accompanied with its genuine and proper symptoms, appear; but when it is exacerbated, either by wrong management or long continuance . . . and Nature is unable to expel it according to her usual way, the symptoms vary considerably from those just described above. For whereas the pain hitherto only affected the feet . . . it now seizes the hands, wrists, elbows, knees and other parts, no less severely that it did the feet before . . . and at length forms stony concretions in the ligaments of the joints, which destroying the skin of the joints, stones not unlike chalk, or crabs' eyes, come in sight and may be picked out with a needle.

These tophi he considered to be due to "undigested gouty matter thrown out around joints in liquid form, and changed to their peculiar hardness by the heat and pain of the joint."

A little later he says, of the chronic phase:

In the last place, before the disease came to such a height, the patient not only enjoyed long intervals between the fits, but likewise had no pain in the limbs and the other parts of the body, all the bodily functions being duly performed. Whereas now his limbs, during the intermission of the disease, are so contracted and disabled that though he can stand, and perhaps walk a little, yet it is very slowly and with great trouble and lameness, so that he scarce seems to move at all . . . the feet in this state of the disease are never quite free of pain.

But besides the above-mentioned symptoms, viz. the pain, lameness, inability to motion of the parts affected . . . the gout breeds the *stone in the Kidneys* in many subjects, either (1) because the patient is obliged to lie long on his back, or (2) because the secretory organs have ceased performing their proper functions, or else (3) because the stone is formed from a part of the same morbific matter; which, however, I do not pretend to determine. And sometimes a suppression of urine, caused by the stone's sticking in the urinary passages, destroys him.

Then comes the famous and much quoted passage:

But what is a consolation to me, and may be so to other *gouty* persons of small fortunes and slender abilities, is that kings, great princes, generals, admirals, philosophers and several other great men have thus lived and died. In short it may, in a more especial manner, be affirmed of this disease that it destroys more rich than poor persons, and more wise men than fools, which seems to demonstrate the justice and strict impartiality of Providence, who abundantly supplied those that want some of the conveniences of life with other advantages, and tempers its profusion to others with equal mixture of evil. So it appears to me universally and absolutely decreed that no man shall enjoy unmixed happiness or misery, but experience both. Since those whom she favors in one way she afflicts in another—a mixture of good and evil pre-eminently adapted to our frail mortality— 'Nihil est ab omni parte beatum'.

As he draws to an end he tells us that:

The *gout* seldom attacks women, and then only the aged, or such as are of a masculine habit of body . . . nor have I hitherto found children or very young persons affected with the *true gout*. Yet I have known some who have felt some slight touches of it before they came to that age, but they were such as were begot by gouty parents. And let this suffice for the history of this disease.

The laity also had their views of the gout. For a distinguished example we find Sir William Temple, in his retirement after a life of diplomatic activity, writing *An Essay on the Cure of the Gout* (1681). From his experience he says of this disease; "I have known a great fleet disabled for two months while the Admiral was neither well enough to exercise, nor sick enough to relinquish, command. I have known two cities of the greatest consequence lost, by the Governors falling ill of it. . . . And I remember one great ruler (the King of France), that confess'd to me, when he fell into one of his usual fits of the gout he was no longer able to bend his mind or thoughts to any publick business, nor give audiences beyond two or three of his own domestics." As Sir William, and others seemed to suggest, gout must be considered not only as inflammation but also as history.

Treatment

Sydenham epitomised his views on the routine treatment of gout as follows: first, to improve the patient's digestion by all possible means; as a preliminary he was prepared sometimes to "clear" the stomach with an emetic and then follow up with a light but adequate diet "as fasting and actual abstinence is not good." If, however, the patient was prepared to forego an evening meal this was to be encouraged. He was also in favour of a non-meat diet occasionally for a few days at a time. "Such patients are better without wine and spirits unless from long habit they cannot digest their food without. Wine with water, or small beer in considerable draughts, to cool and cleanse the kidneys, is best, as simple and crude water is dangerous . . . but young persons may drink it with safety." He advised the addition of anti-scorbutic herbs, such as water-cress, the medicinal prescription of bitters, and the avoidance of salted or spiced foods.

The medicinal treatment of an acute attack entailed bed rest and "the immediate recourse to laudanum, twenty drops of it in a small draught of plague-water. . . . Of all simples the *Peruvian bark* is the best, for a few grains taken morning and evening strengthen and enliven the blood." The Peruvian or Jesuits' bark was the crude form of quinine (*Cinchona*) which had been brought to Europe in 1640 by the Dona Francisca Henriquez de Ribera, fourth Countess of Cinchona, wife of the Viceroy of Peru, and named after her. It is said that Cromwell always refused any proferred relief from "the tainted source of the Popish powder."

Sydenham thought it very important that gouty sufferers should obtain long hours of sleep. Bleeding and purging, the fashionable remedies, he said should only be used moderately, and in selected intractable cases. He had found them "from long and personal experience to do as much mischief in this disease as they do good in others"; although the promotion of sweating in any way was desirable. "The patient must moreover be rendered quiet and easy in his mind, not interested too deeply in studies, not too serious, but cheerful and pleasant."

He strongly recommended regular exercise, "for this strengthens the digestive powers . . . and enables the secretory organs to perform their function of purifying the blood; besides exercise is in some degree preventive of the stone, which an idle and sedentary life generally occasions." But, he warned, "exercise unless it be used daily will do no service."

Finally, he exhorted, of the use of counter-irritants such as blisters, or lighted moxa, fermentations, or lotions:

"Let not external medicines be applied as these will generally drive the disease inward."

He ended his *Treatise*: "And now I have communicated all that I have hitherto discovered concerning the cure of this disease; but if it be objected that there are many specific remedies for the gout, I freely own I know none, and fear that those who boast of such medicines are no wiser than I am." He mused briefly on the credulity of mankind, of all classes and nations in the matter of medical treatment as it is advertised by the quacks and empirics, most of which "heats the parts already disposed to an inflammation, so as to endanger the life of the patient without necessity."

Sydenham evidently subscribed to the contemporary view of many of the laity at this time, that an acute paroxysm of gout will often improve the victim's subsequent general health, as in a letter to a patient of his in Hertfordshire (1687) he wrote: "I could heartyly wish instead of a Merry Christmas that you might have a smart fit of ye gout which would quickly dissipate your other fears, and those symptoms which, if I mistake not, doe naturally desire a discharge . . . I doe advise you to beware of bleeding or purging as diverting this bitter but most effectual remedy, viz., ye gout."

The Master of Manchester Grammar School, Thomas Cogan, in 1584 wrote a small book on popular medicine called *The Haven of Health,* which had a wide circulation and was reprinted into the seventeenth century, in which he gave most of the traditional advice regarding the treatment of gout. Unlike Sydenham, he advocated poultices, which had to be frequently applied by the sufferer himself, and quoted a recommendation of Galen in which an old hard cheese is "cut into pieces and sodden

with the broth of a gammon of a bacone and made in the
manner of a plaster, and laid to the joint where the gout
is. This will break the skin and dissolve those hard knots
which the gout causeth." He also mentioned the value of
wearing an anodyne necklace or one of the various types
of bracelets or rings which were extensively sold for this
purpose, then as now.

Will Atkins, a well-known London quack of the period,
is said to have made a fortune from the sale of such "anodyne" bracelets and rings. He also sold a celebrated "specific for the gout which contains thirty different drugs,
all of which are calculated to ease the complaint. Those
who have no faith in it may keep their money—and their
disease too."

The Honourable Robert Boyle (1627–1691), the gifted
son of the Earl of Cork and one of the founders of the
Royal Society, who invented the air pump and discovered
"Boyle's Law," although not medically qualified wrote
considerably on the subject of gout, from which it is
probable that he also himself suffered. Illustrating the
possibility of curing the acute attack psychologically, by
means of fright, he instanced the case of a cottager known
to him whose hands and feet had been immobilised with
savoury poultices of the sort mentioned by Cogan, and
who had been left in his room alone. "A sow, finding the
door open and attracted by the smell of the poultice, came
to devour it, whereupon the man was put into such a
fright that his pains decreased that very day . . . and
never returned." This was presumably not the type of
danger which had been envisaged by Sydenham, however,
in his repeated warnings against the use of external applications. Heberden also mentioned the virtue in such
cases of: "the sudden alarm of Fire! or of other dangers";
but Dr. Falconer justly observed of this (1788) that

"these matters are rather matters of curiosity than utility, and what we can make no use of in practice."

The remedy with which Sir William Temple tells us he succeeded in curing himself was "the moxa," a small pyramid of a fluffy, cotton-like plant which was placed upon the affected joint and ignited. This was a method imported from the East by the Dutch. It acted presumably as a counter-irritant, like the cautery, and must have required considerable fortitude.

Quackery was rampant, also particularly in the profitable field of syphilis—"the secret disease." Paré, in one of his case histories, succinctly recorded the sufferings of one of his gouty patients and his search for relief, writing: "Neither did he spare any cost or diligence whereby he might be cured of his disease by the help of famous physicians or surgeons; he consulted also with witches, wizards, soothsayers, and charmers, so that he had nothing left unattempted, but all arte was exceeded by the greatnesse of the disease, and then by the emptiness of his purse."

Sydenham's disciples included Sir Hans Sloane, later to become President both of the Royal Society and the Royal College of Physicians; and also one of whom perhaps he was less proud, but who mentions him frequently with affection and respect in his book *The Ancient Physician's Legacy to his Country*, Dr. Thomas Dover (1660–1742), the physician turned buccaneer of the Spanish Main, who introduced his famous "Diaphoretic Compound Ipecacuanha Powder" (Dover's powder) originally as a remedy for the gout. This he was accustomed to prescribe in enormous doses, which led his apothecary to advise the patients to make their will and settle their affairs before taking it. Dover's other chief claim to fame was his discovery of Alexander Selkirk living on the lonely island of Juan Fernandez where he had been marooned for four and a half years. He brought him back and introduced him to Daniel Defoe who wrote up his story as *Robinson Crusoe.*

The seventeenth century introduced the experimental methods of science which in association with the method of inductive reasoning advocated by Sir Francis Bacon, the philosophical Lord Chancellor of England, sounded the death knell of that authoritarianism which had dominated thought since the halcyon days of Greece. Bacon was a great sufferer with the gout, as was his physician, the great William Harvey (1578–1667), the discoverer of the circulation of the blood. Aubrey, in his gossipy *Lives* (published 1813), tells us that "Harvey was much and often troubled with the gout and his way of cure was thus: He would sit with his legs bare if it were frost on the leads of Cockaine House, put them into a pail of water till he was almost dead with cold, then betake himself to the heat of his stove; and so 'twas gone."

The craft of literature also was not immune from this disease, for we are told on no less authority than that of Dr. Samuel Johnson, who suffered severely himself, that the great poet John Milton was tormented by the gout, in addition to his blindness. His doctor, referring to a visit paid to Milton, mentioned that his hands and fingers showed multiple tophi and that the poet had told him that were he free from the pain of the gout his blindness would be tolerable. It has been suggested that inspiration for his vivid description of the torments of Hell in *Paradise Lost* may have derived from his disease.

To summarise: The writings of the great physicians of the seventeenth century, especially those of Sydenham in England and Baillou in France, are so authoritative and often quoted that it is important to assess clearly what actual advances they made in the study of gout and rheumatism during this period. Apart from Sydenham's objective clinical descriptions, it is not really an impressive record. It amounts in its essentials to a more orderly clinical assessment and disinterment of the views of the ancient Greek physicians on this subject; to the rearrangement, along similar lines, of the ancient classification, with gout as a generic term and chronic arthritis in a separate category; and to the important institution of another morbid entity named rheumatism (rheumatic fever), which was still thought to bear some relationship to gout so far as its principal characteristics were concerned. What was referred to as sciatic gout was a synonym for arthritis of the hip joint, and no doubt included infective as well as degenerative and neoplastic entities. Some authors also recognised a category of more superficial non-articular pain of non-gouty origin, "incertae sedis, incerti nominis," which probably corresponds with our modern non-articular syndromes.

CHAPTER VI

Gout in the Eighteenth Century

The eighteenth century, known as the Age of Reason, might also be termed the Golden Age of Gout. Its ravages are well documented in both medical and lay literature and art throughout Europe, and its influence on world history at several important periods can be clearly seen. Everyone who was anybody had it, and those lesser mortals who did not suffer would often simulate what was termed "the honour of the gout." Since the diet of the upper-class Englishman consisted at this time largely of meat protein and port wine, no doubt the mild stress of attaining to a four-bottle handicap would often prove sufficient to establish a congenital tendency. It is on record that in the single year 1733, Sir Robert Walpole, the Prime Minister, spent £8,000 in modern money on wine with his two chief wine merchants, returning 552 dozen empty bottles to one of them. Professor Coste, who was a Privy Councillor as well as physician to the Court of the King of Prussia, wrote (1762): "Les Anglais sont les hommes qui se nourrisent le plus—en excès. Ils ont les meilleurs vivres du monde."

The role of recorded sufferers in Europe reads like a list of the most eminent of their kind. Both France and England were governed by gouty monarchs and first ministers. In England the Secretary of State, Philip Dormer, fourth Earl of Chesterfield, had to resign in 1748 partly to enable him to make the frequent visits to Bath which alone gave him relief. It was of him that Dryden wrote:

> Knots upon his gouty joints appear,
> And chalk is in his crippled fingers found.

Both the Pitts, his successors in office, were grievous sufferers. It was for the same reason that Admiral Lord Howe
had to relinquish command of the British Home Fleet in
1797, and it was this enforced disappearance of "Black
Dick Howe, the Sailor's friend," that precipitated the
tragic and unnecessary mutiny at the Nore.

The literature of the period abounds in references to
the victims of this disease and their sufferings: Smollett
in *Roderick Random, Humphrey Clinker,* and other
works, and Henry Fielding in *Tom Jones;* Laurence
Sterne dedicated his novel *Tristram Shandy* "To the
Right Honourable Mr. Pitt, in the hope that it may help
him to acquire that tranquility of mind that is enjoined
on the gouty sufferer . . . and beguile him of a moment's
pain." The great Dr. Samuel Johnson, after a day of suffering, noted in his diary for 8 December 1765: " 'Tis two
in the morning—I am going to rest with my gout better
and a fire in the chamber—*Fave deus mihi.*" It was no
doubt from similar personal experience that his fellow
poet, Thomson, wrote in *The Castle of Indolence:*

> The sleepless gout here counts the crowing cocks.
> A wolf now gnaws him—now a serpent stings . . .

And again, poor William Cowper, who complained
guiltily one "morning after" of those

> pangs arthritic that infest the toe
> Of libertine excess.

The Honourable John Byng, brother of the British
Admiral who was shot, as Rousseau remarked, "pour
encourager les autres," and author of the eighteenth-cen-

tury *Torrington Diaries,* writing of the benefits which
accrued to the rural population whilst the squires and
their "lady bountiful" wives were resident amongst them,
deplored the fact that: "Since the increase of luxury and
the good turnpike roads, all the gentlemen now have the
gout, and it is found necessary to fly to Bath or to sea-
bathing for relief. . . . How shall the poor exist when
the landlord who protected and supported them is gone
off?"

Across the Atlantic Dr. Benjamin Franklin was writing
his immensely popular *Dialogue with the Gout* in which
he treated of his painful experiences in humourous and
philosophical fashion. He remarked thankfully on his
deathbed that "only three incurable diseases have fallen to
my share, viz., the gout, the stone and old age." John
Wesley, the religious reformer who was also a sufferer and
who dabbled in medicine, wrote a little book which went
through many editions, *Primitive Physick* (1747), in
which he mentioned many of the more homely remedies,
noting after each whether or not he had put it to trial
personally, and the effect.

This apparent association between intellectual ability
and gout, which had first been commented upon by
Thomas Sydenham, was studied by Havelock Ellis (1927),
who wrote that: "It is impossible to regard it as not having
a real association. . . . Genius is not a product of gout,
but it may be that the gouty poison acts as a real stimulus
to intellectual ability and a real aid to intellectual achievement." This hypothesis had, of course, long been a com-
monplace in the case of tuberculosis.

The artists and caricaturists also found in gout a ready
object for their satire. Chief amongst the latter in England
were Rowlandson, Cruikshank, and Gillray, samples of
whose work can be seen in this volume. Sir Alfred Mun-

nings, a contemporary artist-sufferer, thought that it was the ineffective irritability and the unaccustomed helplessness of the often arrogant sufferers with gout that accounted for their treatment as objects of artistic ridicule rather than pity.

Hermann Boerhaave of Leyden (1668–1738), the leading physician in Europe at this time, was also personally interested in the subject of gout. He was described as distinguished in appearance, simple, unassuming, "excessively musical," and the repository of all the medical learning of his time; he fostered in medicine the immensely important development of bedside teaching. He was much addicted to aphorisms and the published volumes of these (1709) were translated into a vast number of languages, including Arabic. As he had noticed that the inflammatory reaction of acute gout never culminated in suppuration, as it did in some other forms of inflammatory arthritis, he conceived the idea that gouty arthritis was determined by mechanical obstruction, due to cold or trauma, of the small capillary vessels which surround the joints; the tophi being the resultant exudate which had become dried out by the heat of the inflamed joint. This hypothesis he transmitted to his distinguished British pupils, William Cullen and Sir John Pringle, and to Van Swieten, physician to the Empress Maria Theresa in Vienna. It later received endorsement from John Latham, physician to the Middlesex Hospital, in his monograph *On Rheumatism and Gout* (1796). Boerhaave also held the curious belief that gout could, in certain circumstances, become contagious, especially to "those who lie much with gouty people"; and Cullen later went to considerable trouble to prove that this was not so. Boerhaave is said to have been consulted by every crowned head in Europe, and when he died he left a great fortune. Many aetiological theories were rife. For Friedrich Hoffmann tartar of wine was "the essential matter of gout," whilst other authorities talked vaguely, but at great length, of such processes as the arrest and decomposition of perspiration.

In England the treatment of gout formed the most remunerative basis of the fashionable medical practices in London and elsewhere at this time. As Sir Richard Blackmore said (1726): "This distemper is not bred in prisons and workhouses, nor engendered in the galley or the mine . . . it is the dissolute and voluptuous indulgence of sensual appetites of the wealthy." Sir Richard, who had pretentions to being a litterateur, was included by Dr. Johnson in his *Lives of the Poets,* although denounced by Pope in his *Dunciad.* Dr. Pelham Warren left a fortune of £100,000, of which he estimated he had gained £30,000 from treating the gout. The other names which are now chiefly remembered in this connection are those of Drs. Heberden, Mead, Radcliffe, Cheyne, and Cadogan—"the Old Masters" of the disease.

Amongst that newly arising class, the scientific chemical physicians, Karl Wilhelm Scheele of Sweden is memorable for his discovery of uric acid in 1776, and William Hyde Wollaston, F.R.S., of London, for demonstrating its presence in a gouty tophus from his own ear, just twenty-one years later. The constituents of tophi had until then been classified as "undigested gouty matter," a description which had seemed adequate to his predecessors.

A small work published in 1793 by Dr. Murray Forbes, entitled *A Treatise upon Gravel and upon Gout,* is of considerable interest as it contains chemical views of a surprisingly modern type. Forbes suggested that as the urine contains uric acid it is probable that the blood must do so also. If this be so, he postulated, it might become precipitated in various parts of the body under certain circumstances. This, he thought, might explain the appearances in acute gout and the tophi in the later stages. It is possible that the book influenced Garrod's work half a century later.

At the beginning of the century appeared Dr. William Musgrave's report, *De Arthritide Symptomatica* (1703), that working with lead could be a cause of gout, and that gonorrhoea could exacerbate it. A further work amplifying these views was published posthumously in 1776, long after Musgrave's death in 1721. Both these observations were confirmed by Dr. Caleb Parry of Bath, and again in the next century by Jean Charcot and Garrod. The two men who perhaps did more than any others to encourage a rational and systematic approach to the subject of gout and its treatment amongst both physicians and the laity, were Dr. William Cadogan and Dr. George Cheyne.

Dr. William Cadogan, F.R.S. (1711–1797), qualified originally at Leyden, but later became physician to the Foundling Hospital in London. William Munk described him as being "of pleasing manners and strong good sense, who by his writing did draw much attention to himself, and paved the way to a lucrative business." His *Dissertation on the Gout* (1771) attracted great attention and went through eleven editions; whilst his sturdy common sense and advocacy of moderation in all things did much to dispel the *mystique* which had long surrounded this disease. The great actor, David Garrick, who was a sufferer, wrote of this: "Dr. C. has written a book lately upon ye gout. It is much admired and certainly has its merit—I was frightened with it for a week." Cadogan maintained that the causes of gout were three in number: "Indolence, Intemperance and Vexation. . . . So it is by the patient's own fault that he is ill," and although he realised that this was sometimes recognised by enlightened physicians, he declared: "Nonetheless, they are afraid to say so, and this talk seems to have been left to me, and I will perform it most sincerely." He concluded: "Let me say that an active and frugal life is a safe preventative, and may be a cure." Cadogan built himself a pleasant country house near London which is now the Hurlingham Club, home of English polo, to which he retired and died at the age of 86.

Dr. George Cheyne (1671–1743) was an Edinburgh graduate who came to London on the advice of his teacher, Pitcairn, and became a Fellow of the Royal Society. After a few years he settled in fashionable practice in Bath "to preach the value of temperance in an intemperate age," although he is described as "a very Falstaff of a man," with much wit, and a double chin. His public reputation as a popular exponent of medical opinion was immense, and his books, including *An Essay on the Nature and Due Method of Treating the Gout* (1720), went rapidly into many editions; seven in the first six years.

In 1760 the newly appointed Professor of Physic in Lausanne, S. A. Tissot, who was treating the historian, Edward Gibbon, the author of *Decline and Fall of the Roman Empire*, there for his gout, published a curious little book entitled *L'Onanisme,* in which he quoted several cases of gout—and many other diseases—as having been caused by this malpractice. In support of this thesis he quoted, with approval, the *Tractatus de Podagra* (1714) of "the late eminent Dr. Clifton Wintringham of York," which had recently been published posthumously by his son, Sir Clifton Wintringham, *Bart.*, F.R.S., chief physician to the Army and to King George III.

Treatment

The method of treatment generally advocated during the eighteenth century was still essentially that employed by the later Greek and Roman physicians, if we except John Abernethy's brusque advice to "live on sixpence a day—and *earn* it." This was the elimination of the "peccant humour" by means of bleeding, purging, and sweating. It is chiefly to the credit of Drs. William Cadogan and George Cheyne that the drastic treatment which was the lot of the sufferer from gout became more rational and civilised towards the end of the century, when a regime of moderation in food, drink, and venery was seriously advocated, together with regular exercise. As the former wrote: "It is one of Nature's strictest laws that one must earn his physical well-being and the pleasure of living by some disbursement of physical exercise or physical toil." Franklin jested at the expense of his fellow sufferers in "Society," who took daily outings in their coaches and called it exercise. Dr. George Cheyne was the first to advocate a completely milk and vegetarian regime for certain cases of gout. This "new venture" attracted much attention, but seems to have been but little practised in that very carnivorous age.

Medicinal therapy was simple and mostly herbal, if we except the many secret "specifics" of the quacks and empirics, some of which contained mineral substances such as antimony, mercury, and arsenic, and were highly dangerous. These were often hawked round the country, and William Donne, writing (1852) of the importance of the eighteenth-century pedlar to the isolated hamlets of rural England, tells us that "He was a great favourite of the village crones for he brought with him the latest powerful medicines for the ague, rheumatism in all its forms, and the Evil." Purgation was coming into fashion again following its ban by Sydenham, but colchicum had dropped out of most of the prescriptions. These generally now contained terrifying mixtures of scammony, colocynth, and aloes, and were expected to achieve for their victims twenty to thirty stools over the two or three days following their administration. Controversy raged around the opiates. Although orthodox opinion was mostly against their use, Sir Richard Blackmore, in *Discourses on the Gout* (1726), expressed the opinion that "opiates are the patient's chief anchor which enables him to ride out the gouty storm"—a view popular amongst sufferers. His favourite prescription was "To take small and strong cinnamon waters, of each an ounce, and liquid laudanum twenty drops, and make of this a draught," which was to be administered several times daily.

Towards the end of the century colchicum was reintroduced by Von Stoerk, the Professor of Medicine in Vienna. He recommended its use principally for the cure of ascites and oedema, however, and failed to produce a satisfactorily standardised preparation. For both of these reasons its use in gout tended to be delayed until the beginning of the next century.

"Specifics"

One of the most interesting of the earlier specifics, from an historical aspect, was the celebrated "Portland powder," which was referred to in many of the writings of the eighteenth century, including the gouty Fielding's *Tom Jones*. The recipe for this was bought for a great sum by the second Duke of Portland and published by him in gratitude for its beneficial effect upon his gout. Its composition was "of equal parts of Birthwort, gentian, germander, ground pine, and the tops and leaves of the lesser centaury. Of this one drachm to be taken every morning, fasting for three months; then ¾ drachm for a further three months," and so on for the whole year. "After this half a drachm must be taken on alternate mornings for a further year; and this will result in cure." It is interesting to note that both Galen and Sydenham had advocated a rather similar mixture of herbal bitters for the same purpose. In the important *Cyclopoedia of the Practice of Medicine* (Ziemmsen), published in England in 1877, Portland powder, as well as other "vegetable bitters," was still advocated! It aroused widespread interest and, although both Cullen and Cadogan thought it dangerous, it was largely employed. Heberden "opined" that "this powder rose to favour too fast and too high to keep its place," but nevertheless thought that it had considerable merit. Probably its ultimate neglect was on account of the large and lengthy dosage required. As late as 1876 Garrod still wrote of it that "I cannot conceive that the exhibition of aromatic bitters in properly selected cases can lead to the evil consequences alluded to by Drs. Cullen and Cadogan, but at the same time caution should be used in administering them." He preferred Boerhaave's small repeated doses of alkaline salines, or lime water.

Another specific which was still used and indeed advocated by some of the leading physicians at this time was Goddard's Drops, which was the first medicine to be patented in Great Britain. It is said to have owed its origins to Dr. Jonathan Goddard, F.R.S., who had been chief physician to Cromwell's Army in the Civil Wars and was later the Gresham Professor of Physic in London. Its composition, which is impressive, is worth repeating as it was sold to Charles II "for the benefit of the Nation" for a large sum.

> Take Humane bones well dryed and broke into bits together with two pounds of viper's flesh. Put them into a retort and distil . . . so will you have a spirit, oyle, and volatile salt. Set it in the earth to digest for three months . . . then separate oyle, which keep for use. If you want it for the gout in any particular limb it is better to make it from the bones of that limb. The dose is six to twelve drops in a glass of Canary Wine; but it has an evil scent.

Dr. John Freind, George II's physician, wrote during his imprisonment in the Tower of London to his celebrated friend Dr. Mead, in somewhat defeatist vein: ". . . but perhaps it were better not to tamper with it [the gout], notwithstanding all these good receipts."

The apparently magical quality of lodestones had always fascinated the learned and the curious, and attempts were made at this time to attribute to them some therapeutic virtue. There is, for example, a report of one "Henry Pelly, Esquire, of Upton, Essex, a lifelong sufferer from the gout, who easily effected a successful cure for his troublesome and painful illness by wearing a very powerful lodestone which he obtained from Golconde round his neck next to his skin." We hear also of other forms of talismen which were to be worn for the same prophylactic purpose. They often consisted in medallions or small phials containing such substances as quicksilver or sulphur, and later iodine; and this practice is still far from extinct.

Spa Treatment

The cult of natural mineral-water therapy had been practised by the Greeks on a carefully regulated system.

It continued under the Romans on an unorganised and semi-religious basis through the Middle Ages, certain holy wells being particularly famed for the cure of certain diseases. To Paracelsus the spas represented nature's laboratories, revealing to men the hidden virtues and powers of the *vix medicatrix naturae*. They came into therapeutic vogue again during the first quarter of the eighteenth century in a more systematic fashion.

Hydrotherapy was re-introduced, chiefly for the treatment of gout, at Buxton, Bath, and other spas in England. It was soon observed that the thermal water at Bath had the property of often producing temporary acute exacerbation of the disease, and it was thought by some that this might prove to be a desirable way of "clearing the air," as long periods of remission often seemed to follow. It was obvious to all that for the use of such powerful waters the best advice was necessary, and many leading physicians, such as Falconer, the friend of John Fothergill, Haygarth, Cheyne, and Parry, soon settled there. In addition to the external and internal prescription of "the waters" they endeavoured also to impose dietetic and alcoholic restrictions, together with regular exercise, upon their fashionable but often recalcitrant patients. William Pitt, the Elder, was the Member of Parliament for Bath and an enthusiastic addict of its waters all his life. The grateful citizens rightly made him an honorary Freeman in 1738.

Horace Walpole, the previous Prime Minister's son, writing from there where he had gone with his friend Grey, the poet, on account of their gout, complained that it bored him, but his consolation was that "Bath is sure of doing some good. I shall take care of myself for fear of being sent hither again." He mentioned that his fellow-patients comprised the majority of the House of Lords, and cynically refers to the place as "the Great National Hospital for Incurables."

The social side of the life of Bath was despotically controlled by the famous Beau Nash, who as self-elected "Master of Ceremonies" was no respecter of persons. He recognised the importance of establishing its reputed medical value on a sound basis, and in conjunction with the Faculty he issued a firm directive which included patients of all ranks—even Royalty. This enjoined that they must appear at 8:30 A.M. sharp, en déshabillé, at the Pump Room, and subsequently "immerse themselves up to the neck as decency requires" daily in the pool before 11:30 A.M.

As most contemporary descriptions of "the cure" are laudatory and somewhat pompously worded, we may quote the more candid opinion expressed in *Humphrey Clinker* by Squire Bramble, who reported to his practitioner as follows:

> I grant that physick is a great mystery in its own nature, and like other mysteries requires a strong gulp of faith to make it go down. . . . Two days ago I went to the Kings' bath, and the first object which met my eyes was a child full of scrofulous ulcers . . . I am now as much afraid of drinking as of bathing, for after a long conversation with the doctor about the construction of the pump and the cistern, it is very far from being clear that the patients in the Pump Room do not swallow the scourings of the bathers.

It was widely believed at this time that gout was incompatible with most other diseases, and sufferers with such differing disorders as "consumption" or melancholia were often sent by their medical advisers to take the waters at Bath in the hope that they might develop an attack of gout, and so overcome their other disabilities.

Spa treatment, however, although widely acclaimed and fashionable, had a severe critic in the celebrated William Heberden (1710–1801), physician to King George III, who said in his famous *Commentaries*: "I have not been able to observe any good in arthritic cases from the external use of these waters, either when the distemper was present or in its absence; on the contrary, it has rather appeared to increase the weakness of the limbs; and sea-bathing has contributed far more to recover the strength of gouty persons." As the result, in due course Brighton and its bathing machines were born.

The Age of Reason gave rise to a growing scepticism in all realms of knowledge and thought, and medicine was not excluded. Towards the end of the century the idea was much canvassed that the evident inability of the physicians to control the paroxysms of the gout might be in accordance with nature's plan to expel the noxious principle itself in this way. This being so, they said, it must be wrong to undergo treatment for this disease, and harmful to check the acute attack, as should the causative humour be driven inwards again it might well attack and inflame the internal viscera, with fatal results. The viewpoint received powerful reinforcement as the result of the sudden death of the second Earl of Buckinghamshire, the Lord Lieutenant of Ireland, after plunging his gouty foot into a pail of ice water. Moreover, as already mentioned, this disease, if maintained, was thought to render the victim permanently free from other more fatal infirmities. Horace Walpole, always in the fashion, expressed this viewpoint in his *Letters*, when he wrote: "I have so good an opinion of the gout that when I am told of an infallible cure I laugh the proposal to scorn and declare that I do not desire to be cured . . . I am serious. . . . I believe the gout a remedy and not a disease, and being so no wonder there is no medicine for it—nor do I desire to be fully cured of a remedy."

Again William Heberden's was the first authoritative voice to condemn this view. He declared (1802): "The dread of being cured of the gout was, and still is, much greater than the dread of having it, in some circles; and the world seems agreed patiently to submit to this tyrant lest a worse should come in its room." He went on to say that "it seems to be the favourite disease of the present age in England. Wished for by those who have it not, and boasted of by those who fancy they have it; though severely lamented by most who in reality suffer its tyranny."

Elsewhere Walpole echoed the complaint of many modern rheumatic sufferers, when he said: "Another plague is that everyone who ever knew anyone who had it is so good as to come with advice, and direct me how to manage it; that is how to have and keep it for a great many years." The evidence of his letters shows him to have been addicted to large doses of Dr. James's antimony powder, however, in spite of his friend Oliver Goldsmith's reputed death from this cause.

Since gout was undoubtedly an occupational hazard of the well-to-do classes in Georgian England, the sufferers were naturally anxious to mitigate the agony of their periodical attacks by as much comfort as possible. In an earlier period Pepys confided to his diary: "To see Sir W. Penn whom I find very ill of the goute sitting in his greate chair, made on purpose for persons sick of that disease, for their ease." Walpole, in his letters, often mentions his "gouty Bootikins," boasting of their efficacy, which he would demonstrate by stamping his gouty foot on the marble hearth to impress his friends who were similarly afflicted. The boots are believed to have reached above the knees and to have been made of oiled silk, padded, and lined with wool, similar to long bedsocks; and, like Harvey, he would also sometimes plunge his legs into ice-cold water before donning them. For more conventional people, however, a well-padded foot-stool at the correct angle was an essential; and in the catalogue issued by the famous cabinet maker, Thomas Hepplewhite, in 1794, is illustrated "the fashionable gouty stool . . . the construction of which being so easily raised or lowered at either end, is particularly useful to the afflicted." His rival, Sheraton, advertised a similar article with the added advantage of "a protective end-piece," whilst the third of the great names of this period, Thomas Chippendale, expressed his willingness to make gout stools to the measurements of the nobility and gentry, in satin-wood upholstered in morocco leather, for a reasonable sum. Chairs on wheels with footrests, which could be self-propelled, were also sold as "gouty chairs." William Pitt, first Earl of Chatham (1708–1778), when Prime Minister, had a gout stool rather like a huge boot built into the front, both of his coach and of the sedan chair in which he was carried from his house in St. James's Square to the House of Commons.

Pitt's gout was of unusual type. His first acute attack occurred at the age of sixteen, and by the age of forty he was almost permanently incapacitated. His sufferings may be considered in some greater detail, as they had ultimately considerable repercussions upon the history of England and the United States.

Pitt had initiated a period of successful struggle with the power of England's old enemy France, both in the Old and New Worlds. But in spite of the national pride in this achievement, the financial cost of his victories was beginning to worry the more timid members of the

Government. They accordingly started to campaign for "Peace at any price," and taking advantage of one of his prolonged attacks of gout they started negotiations with the French. Pitt, hearing of this, had himself carried up to the House of Commons, dressed in black to emphasise his pallor, and with his vast gout boot swathed in rolls of flannel. He was unable to stand on account of the pain, so the House granted him the unique indulgence of a seat during the three and a half hours of his passionate plea against "the eternal enemy" France: "Shall a people that fifteen years ago was the terror of the world now stoop so low as to tell its inveterate enemy, take all we have, only give us peace?" he pleaded. He was, however, defeated and resigned office after the Peace of Paris.

The large bill for the previous Seven Years' War now had to be paid, and as much of its cost had been incurred by defending the American colonists from French conquest, the Stamp Act was passed during Pitt's continued absence due to illness. Under this measure the unwilling colonists were to pay a tax, of an amount to be determined by the Home Ministry, as a contribution. Next year Pitt recovered and succeeded in getting this measure repealed, saying: "The Americans are the sons, not the bastards, of England. As subjects they are entitled to the common right of representation and cannot be bound to pay taxes without their consent. I rejoice that America has resisted. . . . Were I but ten years younger I should spend the remainder of my days in America, which has already given the most brilliant proof of its independent spirit."

He was shortly able to resume office, but under its stresses his gout again struck him down; and during his further enforced absence from this cause his brilliant but unstable colleague, Townshend, treacherously put a heavy colonial duty on tea to raise the extra revenue needed. The result of this was the famous Boston Tea Party in 1773. The Government immediately closed Boston harbour and put the offenders on trial. Pitt's gout went suddenly into remission and he returned to Parliament. By this time, however, things had gone too far for appeasement, and hostilities broke out between the two countries.

That other great gouty character, Benjamin Franklin, now comes upon the scene as official spokesman for the rebellious American colonists. Pitt and Franklin almost wore themselves out trying for weeks together to find some means whereby the two countries might be reconciled. They are also known to have discussed their gouty experiences, as the result of which Franklin is reputed to have said, "Verily Hippocrates hath written much concerning his art . . . but the physician often availeth little, and peradventure fareth he best who boldly taketh the Evil in his own hands and thereof himself prescribeth the cure."

The compromise bill which they eventually evolved, and which had the approval of Jefferson, was put forward by Pitt, but in a crowded House was defeated. Once again his health collapsed; and the War of Independence broke out in full force between England and America. George III now decided that he would direct this himself in the absence of Pitt, whom he greatly disliked, with the result that the world knows.

As the result of his gout and the frustrations induced by the disastrous results of the King's policy, his previous bouts of depression became more severe and Pitt had to spend much of his time in the country, returning only at intervals to voice his protest in the House of Commons. On 8 April 1778, he made his final supreme effort, but it culminated in a fatal stroke, and he was carried insensible from the House of Lords before the end of his speech, to die.

Wallace Graham succinctly commented upon this story: "It would seem a misfortune for England that colchicum was not more widely recognised at that time. It is interesting to speculate whether or not the use of this drug by Pitt's physicians might have prevented the Boston Tea Party and the Battle of Bunker Hill."

So we may wonder today, did America gain independence chiefly on account of the enduring authority of the great Thomas Sydenham, who had opposed in his time a popular purgative prescription containing this drug because it happened to upset his own bowels greatly, and was, as the result, banished from the pharmacopoeias of Europe for over two hundred years?

Looking back over the eighteenth century it would seem that "the demon gout" had established a powerful hold over important members of "the Establishment" of most European countries, and thus exerted considerable influence upon contemporary history. As colchicum had not yet been generally re-introduced into treatment, gout continued to deserve the title conferred upon it by Molière—*La honte des Médecins*.

CHAPTER VII

Gout in the Nineteenth Century and After

Although scientific change was in the air, it was said that the early nineteenth century was the springtime, or heyday, of the gout. As Bywaters (1962) has testified, "tophi like crocuses were bursting everywhere, and 'the honour of gout' was as much a status symbol as a nuclear bomb shelter is now." Tennyson, the great Poet Laureate, was a victim, and his colleague, Mackworth Praed, started one of his poems in apologetic vein: "I've never had the gout, 'tis true. . . ." Every good gouty family had one ancestor who could write on the blackboard with his tophi, even if he were no schoolmaster. The diet of the upper classes in those days was still largely protein and port wine, and the latter cost three shillings a bottle. In 1825, 40,277 tuns were imported, which Halford estimated to be the equivalent of forty thousand cases of gout. Even "poor John Bull in poverty" was portrayed in contemporary caricatures feeding on steak and porter, *vis-à-vis* his French post-revolutionary counterpart "living in luxury" on roots and herbs. William Nesbet, writing in the *London Directory* for 1818, estimated the incidence of gout as being 1:26 amongst the upper-class population, although practically none occurring in the lower orders. It was perhaps fortunate also, as Bywaters pointed out, that the disease was at that time so prominent, both socially and medically, that its abnormal chemical manifestations literally "thrust themselves out," in the words of Sydenham, "like crabs' eyes" for the observation of physicians who were beginning to become interested in the new science of chemistry, which was, as the result of pioneer work by Boyle, Boerhaave, and others, still seeking practical applications primarily in the field of medicine. The old alchemical myths were giving way to the surer foundations of modern chemistry, which may be dated from John Dalton's brilliant statement of the atomic theory in 1808; and the whole field of nature now lay open to the pioneers. Some preliminary triumphs, such as the isolation of uric acid by Karl Scheele, and its discovery in a gouty tophus by Wollaston, predate this era and have already been mentioned. The story of the chemistry of gout was taken further in the course of the new century, chiefly as the result of the demonstration by Sir Alfred Garrod that the blood of sufferers normally contains an excess of this substance. From this he believed it justifiable to postulate that "acute gouty arthritis is an inflammatory reaction to crystals of sodium urate deposited in and about the joint."

From the social aspect gout's prestige was amply maintained in the gouty person of George Augustus Frederick of Hanover, the Prince Regent of Great Britain, later King George IV—"the First Gentleman of Europe"—who referred to gout as "that thorn in the rose of gastronomy." Thackeray, who was an unfriendly critic, asserted that "the Prince was such a powerful toper that six bottles after dinner scarce made a perceptible change in his countenance." Bywaters has shown the large extent to which his life, and thus inevitably the history of his country, was determined by hyperuricaemia at this critical stage in the world's affairs. More intimate details of its ravages are to be found in the pages of Charles Greville's diaries and Creevey's gossipy memoirs of the Regency period. His successor, King William IV, soon after his accession discontinued the age-long custom whereby the monarch had always inspected his troops from horse-back. Greville tells us that "this was on account of the chalk stones in his fingers which rendered it impossible for him to use the reins."

The lesser aristocracy, in whom the gout had been handed down from father to son for centuries, also appreciated its social significance. Dickens introduces us in *Bleak House* to that old county baronet, Sir Leicester Dedlock. During his periods of immobilisation in the ancient oak bedchamber at Chesney Wold he reflects that: "All the Dedlocks in the direct male line through a course of time during and beyond which the memory of man goeth not to the contrary, have had the gout." It had come down through his illustrious line with the plate and the pictures and the family seat in Lincolnshire. And so Sir Leicester was proud to yield up his old family legs periodically to the family disorder, well understanding that "It has for some hundreds of years been understood that we are not to make the [burial] vaults in the Park interesting on more ignoble terms." Readers of Thackeray's *Pendennis* will also remember his elderly friend, the Viscount Colchicum, a dashing old debauchee whose pleasure it was to take selected ladies of the chorus to dine at the Star and Garter in Richmond after the play.

The new scientific undertones did not affect the practical art of medicine, however, for a long time, except for the increasing use of colchicum. Physicians and surgeons continued much as they had always, with their empirical cures and near-mediaeval logic. Such science as they employed resulted from the accurate observational methods which had been made fashionable by Thomas Sydenham towards the end of the seventeenth century. But from now onwards, with the help of the new chemical and other available techniques, these experimental research methods which had been originally sponsored by the Royal Society began to infiltrate medicine, to its great advantage.

The new race of "chemical physicians" included such illustrious names as Justus von Liebig (1803–1873) of Giessen, who started life as an apothecary's assistant, but soon realising the sharp difference between practical pharmacy and scientific chemistry, deserted to academic life and became the father of biochemistry. He considered that the physiological basis of both gout and renal calculus lay in a lack of effective oxidation of the normal products of metabolism which are in excess in such subjects. His remedies, however, were not dissimilar to those of the ancient Greeks and their successors: chiefly abstinence, bitter herbal infusions, and exercise to stimulate the inhalation of as much pure air as possible, to check the retention of carbon dioxide in the system.

In England his disciples included Dr. Henry Bence Jones (1814–1876), the discoverer of the urinary protein which bears his name, who saw in the proper application of hydrotherapy, as currently practised at the German spas, and in particular by "the inspired peasant" Priesnitz at Gräffenburg, the best therapeutic application of this principle. Bence Jones was evidently conscious, however, of additional "fringe benefits" for his patients from this recommended annual trip, as "Some advantage," he says, "is gained from the mere travelling to these baths; passing so many unaccustomed hours in the air causes an increase in the action of the oxygen. Also the sea-sickness decreases the intake of food, and sometimes removes bile." (*Gravel, Calculus and Gout*, 1842.)

Dr. Alexander Ure, of St. Mary's Hospital, also published his "Researches on Gout" in the *London Medical*

Gazette (1844) and recommended benzoate of soda internally, with naphtha applications externally, a combination which he said had the approval of Professor Liebig. He also advocated nicking early tophi with a tenotomy knife and expressing their contents before they hardened, saying that thus they seldom recurred. Many further contributions, some of considerable originality, are to be found in the contemporary literature on this subject, from which we must judge also that the name of Liebig was held little lower than that of the Deity in scientific circles at this time. It is, therefore, surprising to find in a small manuscript notebook compiled by Dr. Matthew Paris for his own use, whilst he was President of the Royal College of Physicians, that after a number of long extracts from Liebig's *Physiological Chemistry,* his final comment was: "All clap-trap!"

Despite the new look which science was giving to general medicine, academic studies did not add much to the knowledge of rheumatology, nor was interest widespread. At the Royal College of Physicians a Goulstonian lecture (1826) and two Croonian lectures (1827 and 1843) were delivered in this field, whilst in 1833, in the first written medical examination to be held in the University of London, candidates were asked: "What are the chief remedies of rheumatism; the circumstances in directing the use of each; and the mode of employing them?"

The chief pioneer in this field was Sir Charles Scudamore (1779–1849). He was himself a sufferer with gout, and, stimulated by the work of John Hunter, he studied his patients objectively and analytically, basing deductions on careful observations and experiments. He initiated crude clinical trials, and even did some valid experiments on dogs. Although his outlook remained completely clinical he made use of those ancillary chemical aids which were becoming available to this new generation of scientific physicians. However, as the result of his investigations he thought that "We have no actual proof even of the existence of uric acid in the body . . . or if present there is no apparent cause why it should not be excreted by the kidneys, the glands obviously designed to separate and excrete saline matter."

Scudamore came of an old Herefordshire family and was the fourth generation to study medicine. He practised as an apothecary in London for ten years before graduating M.D. in Glasgow in 1814 with a thesis entitled *De Arthritide*. His interest in rheumatism was by then well developed, and in 1816 he published *A Treatise on the Nature and Cure of the Gout with Some Observations on Rheumatism*, the first systematic survey of the subject which he dedicated to Matthew Baillie. It was based on his detailed personal observation of about one hundred patients, and proved such a success that a fourth edition had appeared by 1823.

Scudamore considered that previous writers had classified gout in over-elaborate fashion: "As in medicine it is always dangerous to frame distinctions without a difference." He expressed agreement with Latham that three categories were sufficient, namely acute, chronic, and retrocedent. He was a protagonist of the visceral conception of gout, saying that "the inflammatory process will seldom be confined to the joints, but will affect all tissues which are subservient to the function of the joints"; although he avoided the extreme views regarding retrocedent forms which were held by many contemporaries. Regarding this he said: "Dyspepsia and other visceral derangements which commonly occur in a gouty individual are not necessarily dependent upon the gouty state . . . we cannot boast that our knowledge of the intimate nature of disease is sufficient to authorise such conclusions."

He did not believe that gout was invariably hereditary. In an analysis of 523 of his own patients he could conclude an hereditary disposition in 309. Twenty years later Garrod repeated this analysis and reported that of his hospital patients 50 per cent were of hereditary origin; but among his private patients a convincing family history was produced in no less than 75 per cent. During the last twenty years Talbott has reported this finding in two-thirds of all his patients in Buffalo.

Whilst recognising the importance of heredity, therefore, Scudamore believed that an additional precipitating factor was also necessary: "Such as agonising mental stress, or habits sufficiently intemperate to equal such a condition." He commented dryly of the late Prime Minister that: "The late Mr. Pitt and his father both suffered with the gout at an early period of life. The father was a votary of Bacchus; of the son this could not strictly be said; but he was an ardent student." Of the former he also remarked that "he had his existence embittered by the gout, and died of its effects."

Writing of the age of onset of gout he reported that the first attack had occurred between the ages of twenty-five and forty in forty-four of sixty-four patients. He had personally seen no case occurring prior to puberty, an observation with which Garrod agreed; although Gairdner and Trousseau had each reported its occurrence in nurslings. Scudamore believed that gout could not occur after the age of seventy, which led Garrod to publish the case of his patient, the Bishop of Durham, who developed his first attack at the age of ninety-two. They agreed in their belief that the later the initial onset the milder was the course the disease would be likely to run.

Commenting upon the well-observed fact that the initial attack of gout occurs most frequently in the big toe, he reported that in a series of 516 patients this had been so on 341 occasions.

By 1820 Scudamore had been appointed physician to Prince Leopold, and he was knighted by the King during a visit to Dublin in 1829. It was his habit to spend a "busman's holiday" of some weeks each year at Buxton, where he practised in a consulting capacity. On one occasion he analysed the medicinal waters and published the results as a pamphlet (1830).

It was thought that no portrait existed of Scudamore until in 1961 it was learned that Sir William Beechey, R.A., had painted him in 1835, and that the portrait was still in the possession of his descendants. Thus it is through the courtesy of Mr. and Mrs. J. Scudamore that this is reproduced elsewhere in this volume. He was attended on his deathbed by his celebrated pupil and successor, A. E. Garrod.

Sir Alfred Garrod, F.R.S. (1819–1907), although not himself a sufferer, inherited Scudamore's interest in gout and rheumatism, and working along the lines that he had indicated, extended and developed his views. It fell to Garrod to achieve the age-long ambition of his predecessors by identifying uric acid as "the specific morbid humour which inflames all joints in which it enters," which had been postulated as the cause of gout by Hippocrates himself. This he was able to announce in *The Transactions of the Medico-Chirurgical Society* in 1848, as the result of his work at University College Hospital. He wrote: "The blood in gout always contains uric acid in the form of urate of soda, which salt can be obtained from it in a crystalline state." It was, however, a considerable practical drawback that by contemporary chemical analytical methods enough blood had to be drawn from the patient to yield 1,000 grams of serum. It was a practical advance, therefore, when he was able later to describe his famous "uric acid thread test," which was, he said, "an easier mode of ascertaining the presence of uric acid in the blood, which I have been much in the habit of using clinically for many years, and with the results of which I have reason to be well satisfied." Not the least important aspect of "the thread test" was, as he went on to say, that "it is likewise a method which can be readily employed by any medical practitioner, and which has the advantage of requiring the abstraction of only a minute [*sic*] quantity of blood." To perform this test:

> Take from one to two fluid drachms of the serum of blood; to this add ordinary strong acetic acid in the proportions of six minims to each fluid drachm of serum, which causes the evolution of a few bubbles of gas. When the fluids are well mixed introduce one or two end fibres about an inch in length from some linen fabric, which should be depressed with a small glass rod or the point of a pencil. The glass should then be put aside in a cool place until the serum is quite set and almost dry; the mantel-piece in a room of ordinary temperature or a bookcase answer very well, the time varying from thirty-six to sixty hours. Should uric acid be present in the serum in quantities above a certain small amount, noticed below, it will crystallise and will be attracted to the thread and assume forms not unlike that presented by sugar-candy upon a string.

This procedure must have been one of the earliest of bedside clinical diagnostic tests to have been devised and soon achieved world-wide usage. Later Garrod was able to show the presence of urate in the blood even more simply, with the help of the "Murexide test" invented by Dr. William Prout in 1818. Prout was a pioneer of physiological chemistry and one of his principal achievements appears to have been, in the words of the *Diction-*

ary of National Biography, "to show that the excrement
of the boa-constrictor contained 90 per cent uric acid, a
fact of considerable physiological importance." He later
also prepared pure urea for the first time.

With regard to the predisposing causes of gout Garrod
was uncompromising: "There is no truth better established in medicine than the fact that the use of fermented
liquors is the most powerful of all the predisposing causes
of the gout; nay, so powerful that it may be a question
whether gout would ever have been known to mankind
had such beverages not been indulged in." In the last
edition of his book, however, he had mellowed: "It appears," he wrote, "that all causes leading either to an
increased formation of acidity, or its defective elimination and all causes suddenly lowering the nervous system,
have a powerful influence in exciting an attack of gout
in subjects already predisposed to it."

Garrod's work from which I have quoted, *Gout and
Rheumatic Gout* (1859), was a landmark in its field, and
by finally splitting off rheumatoid arthritis from gout,
gave the *coup de grâce* to that ambiguous entity "rheumatic gout." In this work he also recorded his contributions to the basic renal pathology of the disease and the
valid anatomical studies he made in support. It is interesting that he also reports a much lower frequency of
gout and calculus in very hot countries, quoting his
friend, the explorer David Livingstone, as his authority.
His book was translated into a number of other languages
and excited much interest throughout Europe. Garrod
was elected Vice-President of the Royal College of Physicians of London, and in 1890 was appointed Physician
Extraordinary to Queen Victoria, dying in retirement at
the age of eighty-eight.

Another book, which had been published in 1849 and

which went through several influential editions, was *On Gout; Its History, its Causes and its Cure,* by William Gairdner (1793–1867). As he was attached to no hospital Gairdner had ample time for academic study. He also acquired considerable influence, in the words of Munk, from following his profession of domestic and travelling physician to persons of rank and station. Like his contemporary, R. B. Todd (1809–1860), one of the founders of King's College Hospital, whose Croonian lecture (1843) was entitled *Practical Remarks on Gout and Rheumatism,* he postulated a digestive anomaly as the cause of gout, and to some extent endorsed the dietetic advice of Dr. Alexander Haig whose "uric acid-free diet" was fashionable at this time. This may be epitomised in his own words as "Cut out the butcher, and live by the baker, the dairyman and the fruiterer." They believed that as the result of this anomaly the blood became loaded with incomplete products of digestion which precipitated the acute attack. It was Garrod who introduced the view that it was less over-production of uric acid that was the basic factor, than an unwillingness on the part of the kidneys to clear it from the blood normally, a view that was endorsed by Sir Dyce Duckworth in his well-known *Treatise on Gout* (1889).

It was the monumental work of Professor Emil Fischer of Berlin (1852–1919), following that of the Swede, J. J. Berzelius (1774–1848), which first opened the way to further understanding of the structure and synthesis of the proteins of the purine group. For this he was awarded the Nobel Prize in 1902. His work led to the development of micro-methods of blood analysis and the use of isotopic labelling, all of which greatly increased our knowledge and control of the biochemical defects which constitute the gouty and hyperuric states, and the various aberrations associated with its metabolism. It was also discovered that the body can synthesise purine materials from simple basic elements. The introduction of Folin's simple colometric method of estimating uric acid in the blood (1913) also led to routine studies in this disease, and to the interesting finding that many relatives of gouty sufferers who may themselves never manifest any outward signs of the disease, will nevertheless be discovered to be hyperuricaemic.

In 1890 Sir Archibald Garrod, who like his father had been physician to the West London Hospital before moving on to the staff at St. Bartholomew's Hospital, published his *Treatise on Rheumatism and Rheumatoid Arthritis* in which he analysed further many of the case records of Sir Alfred's gouty patients. These are still of considerable interest, although he made no notable personal contribution to the subject.

In 1905, after the use of X-rays had become general, it was pointed out by Dr. T. S. P. Strangeways that in gout urates were often deposited within the cortex of bones, giving rise to those cyst-like "punched out areas" which are now regarded as characteristic findings.

Treatment

The treatment of gout for two-thirds of the nineteenth century did not show much basic change from that of the eighteenth, except for the empirical introduction of colchicum. Even this innovation was not accepted by all, and it seems curious that the great French physician, Trousseau, denounced colchicum until the end of his life; he also wrote that the then fashionable use of mineral waters was almost equally dangerous. Scudamore, whilst approving the use of colchicum, wisely publicised its side effects. In 1820, with progress in chemistry, Pellétier and

Caventou had been able to isolate from it the alkaloid colchicine, and this was produced in crystalline form by Houdé in 1884. This development of newer drugs facilitated rapid control of the acute attack of this ancient disease and so rendered treatment more effective and predictable, and dosage more accurate. The use of external remedies continued to be suspect as it was thought that in some way they tended to "fix the inflammation" in the affected joints.

With the growing understanding of the need for restricting purines and fat the dietetic treatment of gout became less empirical, and the discovery that tea and coffee are methylated purines which do not form uric acid in the body brought comfort to many who had suffered their deprivation unwillingly. It is probably to this period that the belief in fresh lemon juice as a sovereign remedy for gout and rheumatism may be assigned, as Sir William Roberts (1830–1899) opined that as it was "constituted of pure citric acid and some salts of lime and potash, the latter should act favourably in neutralising the rheumatic poison." In this he was supported by his colleague, G. O. Rees, F.R.S., of Guy's Hospital. The importance of a low meat diet was well recognised, and Admiral Nelson, when he was stationed at Malta and began to have frequent attacks of gout, was advised to abstain from all animal food and took only vegetables, milk, and water for many months. His gout cleared up, as did also the dyspepsia from which he had suffered for years.

The specific sensitivity of some individuals to certain types of foods as well as drink was discovered and studied. This knowledge soon became common amongst the laity, and we find a significant entry in the Reverend Sydney Smith's amusing diary, following his first attack of gout in

1829: "When now I feel a pang I say to my body I know what this is for. I know what you mean! I understand the hint." In his case plums and marzipan appear to have been prime *agents provocateurs*. It was he who wittily stated that "the only enemy that I do not wish to see at my feet is the gout." His practical appraisement of another dietetic facet should be quoted: "Proper cooking will have much to do with remedial measures," he said. "The sufferer must also enter into a solemn compact with his stomach to relinquish all serious flirting with the *sirens* of the kitchen and the *houris* of the wine cellar"— a regime he referred to as "stomatic monasticism."

Wines

Some remarks upon this controversial subject, which has attracted the interest of every generation of sufferers and their physicians, may not be out of place here. From the time of the legendary invention of champagne in 1718 by Dom Pérignon, a Benedictine monk of Rheims, there appears to have been almost unanimous agreement that this wine will precipitate attacks of gout. An important early exception to this opinion was presented personally by the distinguished Professor of Medicine at Trinity College, Dublin, Sir Edward Barry, F.R.S., the author of *The Wines of the Ancients and the Analogy between Them and the Modern Wines* (1775). From the time of "the glorious Revolution" of 1688 it became customary to fortify the French wines in general use with brandy, and for that reason, according to Sir William Temple, the incidence of gout rose greatly. There was a contemporary jingle which started: "Burgundy rose! Burgundy rose! 'Tis a very bad thing at the tip of our toes!", a sentiment with which Sir Charles Scudamore expressed agreement in more dignified terms. He said

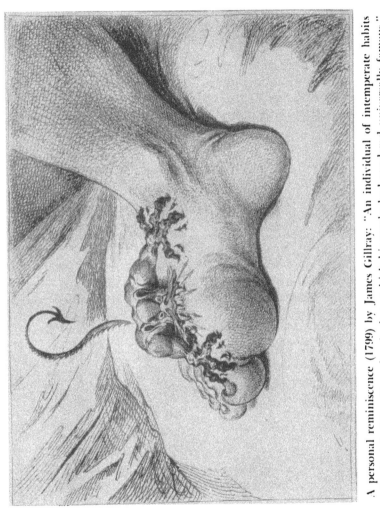

A personal reminiscence (1799) by James Gillray: "An individual of intemperate habits who died in Miss Humphrey's shop, which his works had rendered universally famous."

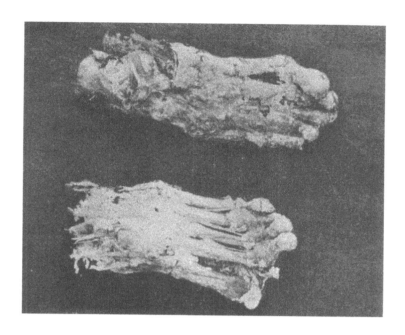

True gout in the great toes of an early Christian. The hands were also affected. These specimens were destroyed in 1941 when the Royal College of Surgeons of England was bombed. Illustration from *Archaeological Survey of Nubia* (1908) by courtesy of the President.

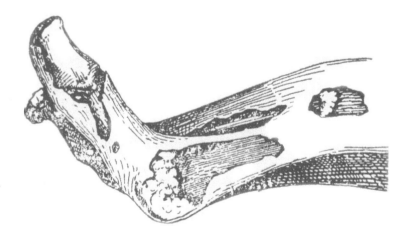

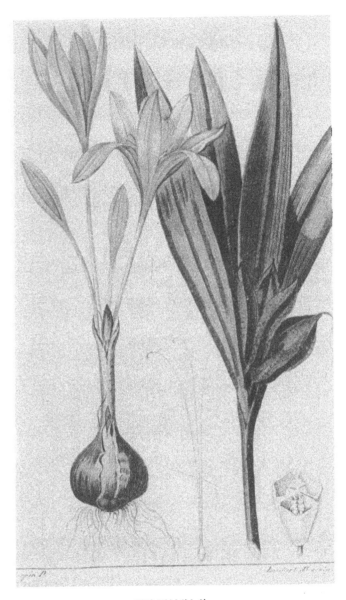

COLCHIQUE.

Colchicum, or the Meadow Saffron. From a French herbal
(F. Panckouke, 1814).

Podagrammisch
Trostbüchlein

Innhaltend

Zwo artlicher Schuz = Reden von herliche
ankonft, geschlecht, Hofhaltung, Nuzbarkait vn
tifgesuchtem lob des Hochgeehrten, Glidermäch
tigen vnd zarten Fräuleins PODAGRA.

Nun erstmals

zu kizeligem trost vnd ergezung anbächtiger Pfoten
grammischer personen, oder Handkrämpfigen vnd Fus
verstrickten kämpfern lustig vnd wacker (wie ain Hun
auf dem Lotterbett) bossirt vnd publicirt

Durch
Hultrich Ellopocleron.

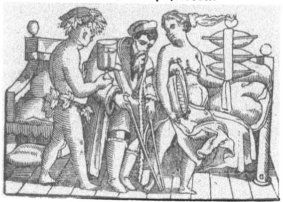

Anno **M. D. LXXVII.**

Title page of the earliest printed book on gout (Johann Fischrt. 1577).

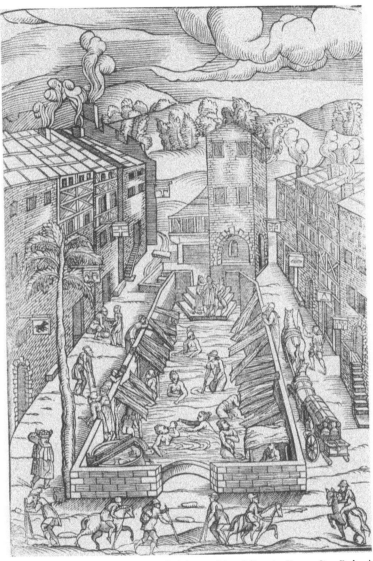

Spa treatment for gout and arthritis (at Plombières). From *De Balneis* (1553).

Sydenham's notebook; in possession of the Royal College of Physiciar
The top portion is in his own writing. By permission of the Presider

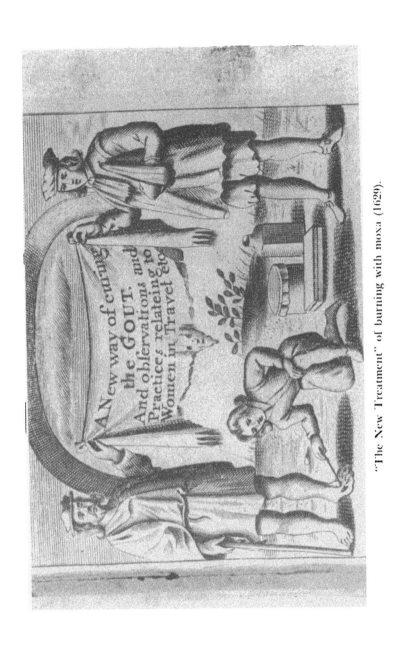

A New way of cureing
the GOUT.
And obſervations and
Practiceſ relateing to
Women in Travel &tc

"The New Treatment" of burning with moxa (1629).

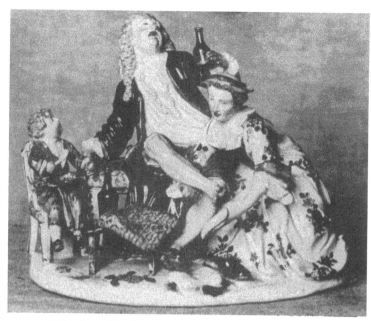

"The Joys of Podagra." Meissen porcelain group (1745).

"A Chair for the Gout" (c. 1800).

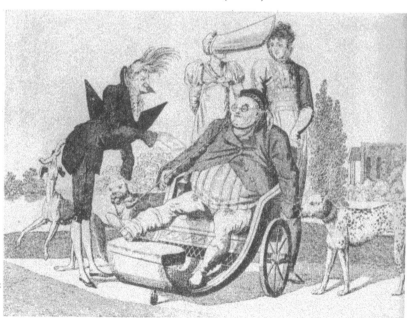

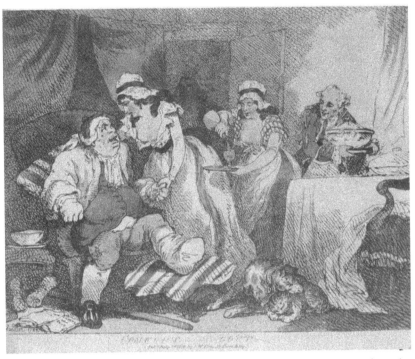

"Comfort in the Gout" (J. Rowlandson. 1785). A reaction to Cadogan's "Austerity Regime."

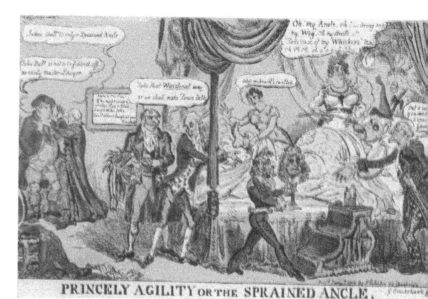

PRINCELY AGILITY or the SPRAINED ANCLE.

The Prince Regent's first attack of the gout, 13 November 1811.

The machine devised for the Regent at his Chinese Pavilion at Brighton: "To enable him in some degree to enjoy the benefit of air and exercise" (*Times*, March 1818). Cartoons by George Cruikshank. Colour plates by courtesy of the *Annals of the Rheumatic Diseases*, London.

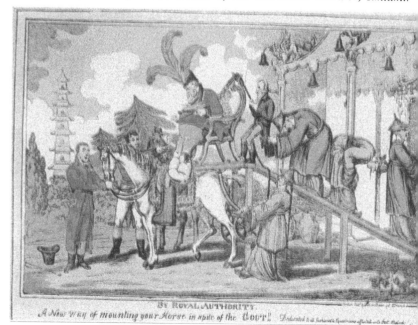

BY ROYAL AUTHORITY.
A New Way of mounting your Horse in spite of the GOUT!!

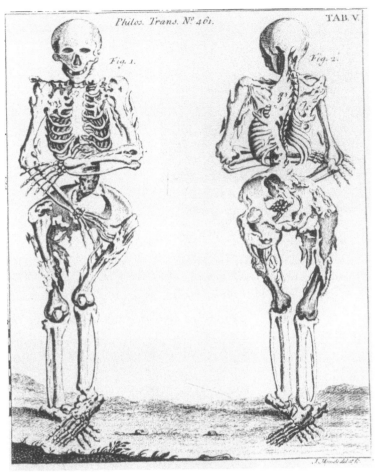

Spondylitic spine, described by the Bishop of Cork to the Royal Society of London, 1741.

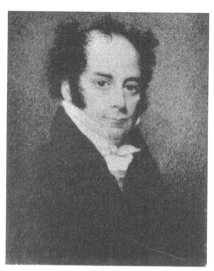

Sir Charles Scudamore (1788–1836), historian, and the father of rheumatology.

Sir Alfred Garrod, F.R.S. (1819–1907).

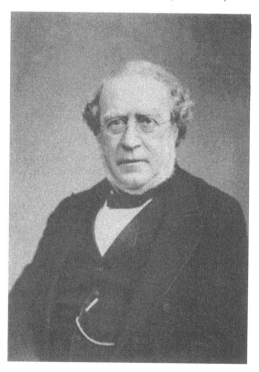

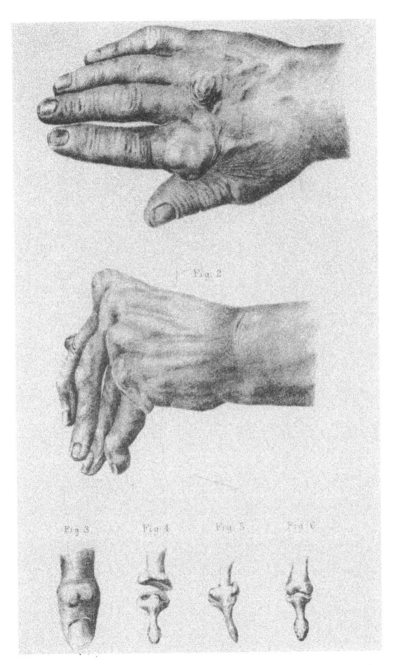

Fig. 2

Fig. 3   Fig. 4   Fig. 5   Fig. 6

Charcot's drawings (1868) of: (1) a gouty hand showing a large tophus:
(2) rheumatoid arthritis; (3) "The anatomy of Heberden's nodosities."

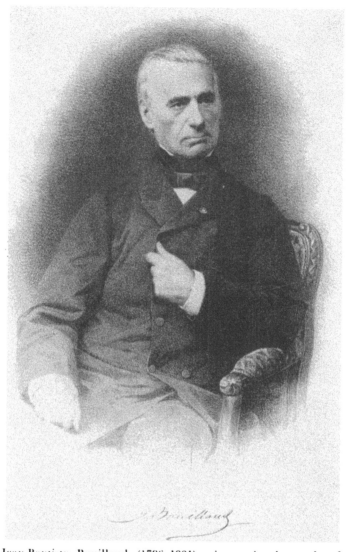

Jean-Baptiste Bouillaud (1796–1881), pioneer in the study of rheumatic fever, "Bouillaud's Disease."

A

TREATISE

on

CHRONIC RHEUMATIC ARTHRITIS,

or

RHEUMATIC GOUT.

PART I.

THE DISEASE CONSIDERED GENERALLY.

CHAPTER I.

HISTORY OF THE DISEASE.

THE disease which I am about to describe in the following pages has been already adverted to by medical writers, who have given to it different names, as it presented itself in different regions of the body. Thus, when the wrists, hands, and feet have been affected by it, the disease has been denominated "Rheumatic Gout," but when the shoulder, elbow, or knee-joints have been either singly or simultaneously engaged, it has generally been named "Chronic Rheumatism."

It is well known that this same malady sometimes fixes itself in the various structures which enter into the composition of the hip-joint, producing a chronic

B

The opening page of Robert Adams' *Treatise on Chronic Rheumatic Arthritis* (1857).

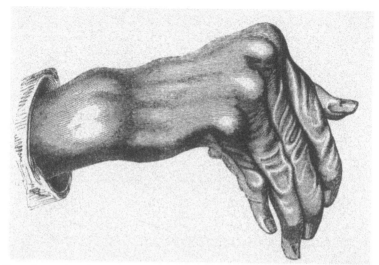

Drawings of a rheumatoid hand: (1) disease of eleven years' duratior
(2) post-mortem appearance. From Robert Adams (1857

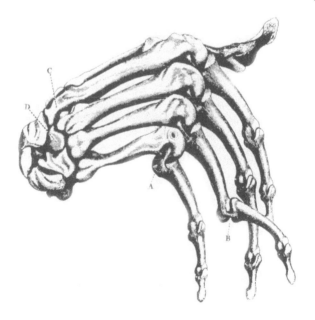

"Burgundy is, of all wines, the most certain fuel to the gout."

In 1703 gouty Queen Anne concluded the Treaty of Methuen, whereby port wine was substituted for the French wines. This was widely welcomed "as an antidote to the damp climate and fogs of England, the inhabitants being at that time unaware of the canker that lurks in every glass for the gouty subject." Dr. F. W. Pavy's opinion that "nothing is more potent than port-wine in leading to the production of gout," was expressed forcefully in his Harveian Oration (1886).

Good claret and the white German wines of the Rhine and the Mosel were thought during the nineteenth century to be comparatively innocuous, and were even sometimes recommended as "morale raisers" by such men as Scudamore and Sir Thomas Watson. All malt liquors were, however, rightly proscribed, as were sherry and madeira wine. Of the latter Lowell wrote: "I call my gout the unearned increment from my grandfather's madeira, and think how excellent it must have been—I sip it from the bin of fancy, and wish he had left to me the cause instead of the effect."

It had been remarked by observers as far back as Galen that in districts where unfermented cider was largely consumed, gout seemed to be rare; thus it came to be looked upon as a preventive. It was the practical Dr. Heberden who pointed out that "It might be that this drink is chiefly used by those who lead simple and laborious lives and earn their daily bread by the sweat of their brow. Were the peasants of Devonshire or Brittany to inherit a generous fortune and lapse into luxury," he believed it would be a question "whether cider would not then prove a dangerous draught for the potential victim of this disease." Garrod gave it as his opinion that "taking different varieties of alcoholic beverages at one meal is greatly more injurious to the gouty sufferer than the same amount of any one kind."

The modern view was perhaps first formulated by Sir Dyce Duckworth (1889) who deprecated the consumption by gouty sufferers of malted or fermented liquors of all sorts; but if drink were really necessary they should confine themselves to well-diluted whisky in moderation. Of this he comments further: "It is useless to urge total abstinence on one who has been an immoderate drinker all his life. He may perhaps acquiesce in moderation, but will kick at deprivation. Such a patient should, however, at least be an abstainer between meals—not merely between drinks."

Physical exercise during this century was once again highly regarded, and Sydenham's words were recalled: "This is as sovereign a cure as we shall see." Scudamore pointed this moral by his observation that when he graduated in Glasgow (1814) gout was almost unknown there. This he attributed to the fact that nearly all the inhabitants of this rich city walked constantly as there were but five hackney carriages and twenty private conveyances within its wide boundary. Trousseau succinctly expressed the desirability of combining physical exercise with mental relaxation with his aphorism: "Fatiguez la bête, mais reposez la tête."

In the chronic phase of gout Garrod advocated the use of potassium iodide and guaiacum by mouth, together with simple alkaline salines "on account of their action in alleviating affections of fibrous tissues." In 1843 Dr. Andrew Ure, F.R.S., had reported in *The Pharmaceutical Journal* his success in dissolving a uric acid calculus in a solution of lithium carbonate. Following this line Garrod introduced the oral use of lithia salts for gout in

1858. The object was to increase the rate of excretion of uric acid by putting it into solution. The initial apparent success of this treatment sufficed to introduce both the carbonate and citrate of lithia into the first edition of the *British Pharmacopoeia* in 1864, where they remained until recently.

Most medical men, however, had their own particular fads and fancies. For instance Dr. James Carrick Moore, long-lived brother to the hero of Corunna, wrote to "his eminent friend" Sir Astley Cooper, the King's Surgeon, on 13 February 1837: "I regret to hear you are attacked with the gout which is torture to the stoutest. Don't mind what Sir Charles [Bell] or Dr. Bright recommend, but take my sapient council: Every night swallow 20 minims of vinum veratri in a glass of weak hot wine whey: and half a drachm of magnesia in ginger tea in the morning. If you obey me you will soon be well. I remain, dear Sir Astley, your volunteer doctor, J. C. Moore."

Various highly specialised forms of diet were also introduced. Of these Dr. Alexander Haig's "uric acid free diet" was the most celebrated. This aimed to increase the alkalinity of the blood so that uric acid would be retained in suspension and excreted. Much was to be omitted, including meat, fish, eggs, and tea, coffee, and cocoa.

For the long-term control and management of gouty arthritis it was, however, necessary to find substances capable of influencing the level of the uric acid in the circulating blood. The first of these, cinchopen, which was generally known as "atophan," had been discovered and synthesised in 1887 by Doebnev and Giesecke, and was introduced as a uricosuric agent for long-term treatment in 1911 by Weintraud of Berlin. This served its purpose for a time, despite its often dangerous side effects. It was also discovered that salicylates, if given in very large doses, would serve the same purpose of preventing the level of uric acid in the blood climbing to an height at which an acute attack would be triggered off, but patients seldom were able to tolerate these in sufficient quantity indefinitely. The fact that it was now possible to control the level of uric acid in the blood, however, constituted a great advance in the possibility of controlling the disease.

It was only in 1948, exactly one hundred years after uric acid had been detected as the *fons et origo* of gout, that the chemical discoveries already chronicled began to bear really satisfactory fruit from the patients' point of view. In this year, as a by-product of penicillin research, carinamide was discovered. This and its pharmaceutical progeny were destined to be effective, safe, uricosuric agents, and within a few years, introduced into medical practice for this purpose, replacing atophan in an improved and non-toxic form known as probenecid (1951). Further synthetic variants on this substance are still introduced at frequent intervals, which all have the power of inducing in the body a negative urate balance, either by influencing the production of uric acid or, as is more likely, by stimulating the kidneys to part with it more readily.

It had always been suspected that gout might have differing origins. It is only during this twentieth century, however, that primary or hereditary gout has been clearly differentiated from a number of secondary types which may result from other kinds of diseases such as polycythaemia, certain anaemias, and affections of the haemopoietic system as well as the ingestion of certain modern drugs. Gout due to such causes must naturally receive the treatment appropriate to its origin.

The disease still keeps its ultimate secrets, although

increasing knowledge of its chemical processes is being gained. Some of these are tending to complicate the simple and satisfactory conception revealed by Garrod. It seems that uric acid is no longer all! It is becoming increasingly evident, however, that gout is the end product of a disordered body metabolism, which is often genetically acquired, and although we are rapidly learning to understand this, it would seem unlikely that we shall be able to rectify it. We are, however, justified in the optimistic assumption that we shall very shortly be able to manage the various manifestations of gout, both acute and chronic, to our satisfaction.

It is humiliating, after writing this last paragraph, to note a news item in the *Times* of London, headed: "Pilot's Gout Stops Air Service." This records that flights between Cornwall and the Isles of Scilly had to be suspended during April because "The pilot was smitten with gout. This was the first interruption of this service since 1937." Such a situation seems unlikely to recur frequently in the future, however.

We have not yet reached the end of the fascinating story of gout. There is a great deal more that we shall learn, and the rate of advance recorded in this chapter renders it probable that this further progress will be accomplished within the next few years.

CHAPTER VIII

Acute Rheumatism and Chorea

Acute Rheumatism or Rheumatic Fever

The modern conception of acute rheumatism, or rheumatic fever, as an important constitutional disease of infective origin which constitutes a major scourge of childhood and a formidable cause of heart disease, was only arrived at very gradually.

The history of this disease can be divided into four main periods. The first is that of the ancient Greeks, who separated it from gout as a clinical variant. The second began in 1642 with that posthumous publication of the great French physician, Guillaume de Baillou, in which the word rheumatism was first used in its modern sense. The third great advance was marked by the realisation by David Pitcairn (1788) that acute rheumatism is more than merely a disease of the joints but can equally affect the heart and so be an important cause of death amongst the young. Finally, with the publication in 1836 of Jean-Baptiste Bouillaud's great work *Nouvelles Recherches sur le Rhumatisme Articulaire*, there was established the fundamental basis upon which modern ideas of the disease were based.

The first period

This spanned only the life of Hippocrates who based his conclusions on practical observation, and who may have recognised acute rheumatism as a separate entity.

Quite possibly, however, he still regarded it as a clinical variant of gout. He declared: "The joints become swollen and painful. The disease assumes an acute form and the pains, varyingly sharp, wander first from one articulation and later to another . . . the disease is short and acute, but not fatal. Usually it attacks young people rather than the aged." The immediate followers of Hippocrates seem to have ignored this distinction, perhaps because acute rheumatism was rare in Greece although indigenous in Rome under the name of "morbus articularis." At any rate, throughout the Middle Ages most disease syndromes which affected the joints were grouped under the generic term "arthritis," and were regarded merely as differing forms of gout, the arthritic prototype with which they were most familiar.

During the Renaissance we find the accomplished Italian physician, Jerome Cardan (1501–1576), who, in addition to his many medical works, wrote widely on such erudite subjects as the solution of cubic equations in algebra, why the stars twinkle, how to catch mice, and how to avoid sea-sickness, and the great humanist, Jean Fernel (1497–1558) in France, both resuscitating the Hippocratic idea of acute rheumatism as a clinical entity quite independent of gout.

Realdo Colombo, in his *De Re Anatomica* (1559), described the post-mortem examination he carried out on a cardinal who had died at the early age of forty: "I saw a hard tumour, the size of an egg, in the left ventricle of the heart." This, Professor O'Malley considers, was probably an organised thrombus developing from the vegetations of rheumatic endocarditis, and so the first recorded reference to the pathological sequelae of this disease.

The second period

Guillaume de Baillou (1538–1616) is generally considered as the "Father of Rheumatism," as it was he who first used this word in its modern sense of an acute polyarthritis which has no connection with gout. He classified diseases of the joints into (1) podagra, (2) acute and chronic polyarthritis, which he thought to be clinical variants of gout, and (3) rheumatism. The word "rheumatism" had been used by the ancients in the sense of something flowing through the body, causing disease and pain wherever it settled. It had, however, become in course of time merely a loose, lay expression implying pain of obscure origin, and it was Baillou who adapted it to imply a special form of acute arthritis. As de Sèze observed: "He took the name from vulgar use, and the theory from Galen."

Baillou wrote: "The method whereby this affliction attacks is falsely called catarrhal, which implies a distillation of humours flowing down from the head. It seems better to speak of it as Rheumatism . . . and although arthritis occurs in a single part, rheumatism invades the whole body with pain, swellings and a keen sense of heat." By this he evidently meant that rheumatism is to the whole body what gout is to individual joints. He went on to say, in description of the attack:

> The joints are wracked with pain so that neither foot, hand nor finger can be moved without pain and protest . . . the affected parts are found to be very hot. The pain becomes exacerbated at night . . . the arthritic pains are recurrent, and the patient cannot sleep.

He warned also that "Those who suffer two or three times from rheumatism, unless they take care of themselves, can scarcely hope to escape chronic arthritis."

Baillou enunciated his views within the walls of the
Faculty of Medicine in Paris, of which he was a revered
member, but they were little known to the outside
world, however, until his nephew published his lecture
notes of 1591 as the celebrated *Liber de Rhumatismo*
(1642). Although primarily a scholar, such was Baillou's
fame that despite his refusal King Henry IV appointed
him physician to his son, the dauphin. He wrote much
and was the first to describe whooping cough; whilst his
study of environmental factors which influence disease
have led to his being termed "the first epidemiologist of
modern times." His biographer, Moreau, tells us that
"he filled all the world with admiration and excited the
envy of some, although no one was forthcoming enough
to claim to share with him the glory." All the same his
own claim that acute rheumatism had never, until his
time, been recognised is, as we have seen, not strictly
true.

The first really satisfactory clinical description of acute
rheumatism was given some years later by Thomas Sydenham. In spite of Baillou's work most seventeenth-century
physicians still persisted in regarding rheumatism and
gout as variants of the same disease. Sydenham, however,
a lifelong victim of the gout, recognised that they were
quite different diseases, each with characteristic clinical
features easily distinguishable from other joint affections.

He portrayed the onset of a typical attack of rheumatism in the following well-known words:

> The disease comes on at any time, but especially in the
> Autumn, and chiefly seizes those that are in the young
> flower of their Age . . . It begins with shivering and shak-
> ing, and presently heat, restlessness and thirst; and other
> symptoms which accompany Fever. After a day or two, and
> sometimes sooner, the Patient is troubled with a violent

> Pain, sometimes in this, sometimes in that Joint; in the
> Wrist and Shoulders, but most commonly in the Knees; it
> now and then changes places, and seizes elsewhere, leaving
> some redness and swelling in the Part it last possessed. . . .
> When this Disease is not accompanied with a Fever it is
> often taken for the Gout though it differs essentially from
> that, as plainly appears to anyone that well considers both
> Diseases.

Scurvy was an affliction which was common in England
at that time. During the winter most of the population
perforce fed on salted foods and even at other times fruit
and vegetables were not universally much eaten. Sydenham recommended the addition of "scurvy grass" and
water-cress to the diet of rheumatic patients, and so was
able to resolve the confusion which soon arose owing
to the similarity of the symptoms of subacute rheumatism and scurvy in many cases.

The great Dutch physician, Hermann Boerhaave
(1668–1738), the "Batavian Hippocrates," wrote an excellent description of the disease based upon that of Sydenham whom he much admired. He began by saying:

> There is a disease ally'd to the Gout and the Scurvy which
> is very common in England and call'd Rheumatism. It
> begins with a continual Fever, creates a most terrible tear-
> ing Pain, increasing cruelly upon the least Motion, long
> continued and fixed in one Place, obsessing the joints of
> any Limb, but most particularly troublesome to the Knee,
> Loins and Rump-bone, excruciating and invading some-
> times the Brain, Lungs and Bowels, with a swelling and
> redness of the Place, and going off and returning by fits.

It has often been thought that Boerhaave was describing
his own experiences in his first attack of acute rheumatism, in 1721, a recurrence of which forced him ultimately to retire from practice.

Visceral Involvement. The chief importance of Boerhaave's work was his recognition of visceral involvement in the course of this disease which had previously been regarded purely as one affecting the joints. It was his pupils Von Stoerk and Van Swieten, however, who first appreciated its real importance and supported these observations by post-mortem examinations. The former, in his *De Febre Arthritica* (1762), declared in describing a case seen by him: "The rheumatic poison which had seized the joints of the hands and feet then dispersed through the whole body . . . afterwards the breast was affected, attended with a difficult respiration that shortly threatened suffocation." Van Swieten said elsewhere: "While the rheumatism attacks only the joints it is rarely fatal; but when it seizes the brain or lungs it is highly dangerous." He did not actually mention cardiac involvement, but this might perhaps be inferred from a clinical report in which he noted, in his *Commentaries upon Boerhaave's Aphorisms* (1776), that: "Sometimes when the pain in the limbs ceases there arises an anxiety in the breast, a palpitation of the heart, and an intermitting pulse."

William Cullen of Edinburgh (1712–1790), another of Boerhaave's distinguished pupils, also gave a good account of acute rheumatic polyarthritis in his famous *First Lines of the Practice of Physic* (1776). Following the lead of Sauvages he divided the disease into "two species, the one named the acute, the other the chronic rheumatism . . . although the limits between the acute and chronic rheumatisms are not always exactly marked." He did not refer anywhere to visceral involvement, but suggested that lumbago and sciatica might result from this disease, implicating the lumbar vertebrae and the hip joint respectively.

His views on the aetiology of rheumatic fever were

personal and curious. A cold environment, he thought, would cause constriction of the blood vessels which nourished the joints. The body, with the help of its native "nervous energy," would endeavour to overcome this vascular obstruction, but would cause a local inflammatory reaction by so doing. If this were prolonged it would pass over into a generalised inflammation of the blood-stream which thus produced the fever.

It is probable that many acute and chronic infective conditions were being classified indiscriminately under the new nosological headings, which included acute rheumatism. Cullen seems to have recognised this as he remarked of the "true" acute rheumatism that "though it has so much of the nature of other phlegmasiae, it differs from all those hitherto mentioned in this, that it is not liable to terminate in suppuration. This almost never happens in rheumatism." As the result of Cullen's interest in rheumatology the subject became the object of serious study in Scotland for the first time, and between 1775 and 1827 no less than forty-two academic theses for the M.D. degree were approved by the University of Edinburgh, and another thirty between 1800 and 1833, some on acute and some on chronic rheumatism.

It was William Heberden who was one of the first to point out that acute rheumatism is largely a disease of childhood. In his *Commentaries* (1802) he said: "The rheumatism has appeared so early as in a child only four years old. I have seen several afflicted with it at the age of nine years; in which it differs from the gout, which I have never observed before the years of puberty."

The third period

The increasing practice of post-mortem examination in the eighteenth century led to great improvement in

pathological knowledge. It was thus that the close association between cardiac pathology and rheumatism was
finally appreciated.

It seems probable that rheumatic heart disease was
recognised as a clinical entity by several of the leading
physicians of the time, although they failed to leave
written evidence of this fact. It was only a casual paragraph in the second edition of Matthew Baillie's *Morbid
Anatomy* (1797) which secured for Dr. David Pitcairn of
St. Bartholomew's Hospital the priority (1788) in this
matter. Baillie wrote: "The causes which produce a
morbid growth of the heart are but little known, one of
them would seem to be rheumatism attacking this organ."
A note at the bottom of the page adds: "Dr. Pitcairn has
observed this in several cases." This was the first time
that the close causal relationship of rheumatism to organic
heart disease was commented upon in print. Had it not
been for the unfortunate loss of the manuscript of the
paper which Edward Jenner, the celebrated exponent of
vaccination, delivered to the Gloucestershire Medical
Society on 29 July 1789, at the Fleece Inn at Radborough,
entitled *Remarks on a Disease of the Heart following
Acute Rheumatism, Illustrated by Dissection,* it would
probably have been he who would officially have received
priority for this observation.

It is not known what Jenner's dissection showed, but
presumably some lesion of the valves. This became recognised as a pathological sequel to endocarditis after Baillie's description (1797) of a case of "ossification of the
valves" after heart disease in the following terms: "The
valvular apparatus between the auricles and ventricles
is liable to the formation of bony and earthy matter.
. . . What this depends upon it is very difficult to determine . . . this apparatus is also occasionally thickened,

having lost all its transparency and having an opaque
white colour."

Dr. John Haygarth (1740–1827) of Bath wrote *A Clinical History of Acute Rheumatism* (1805), which was the
first monograph on this subject and is now excessively
rare. He noted, amongst other points, that the disease
tends to attack more males than females, and affects its
victims most frequently between the ages of fifteen and
twenty years; but, curiously, he does not mention any
association between rheumatism and the heart. Equally
unexpected is his history of an analogy between the ague
(malaria) and acute rheumatism, which led him strongly
to advocate "the bark" (quinine) for the treatment of
both. But science crept in when he based clinical and
therapeutic conclusions upon "a study of 170 personally
and carefully observed cases." This section, as Bywaters
has pointed out, is couched in quite modern statistical
form, paying due regard to criteria of diagnosis and improvement.

By the beginning of the nineteenth century the close
association between acute rheumatism and *morbus cordis*
had become evident to the majority of medical men in
Europe; and the death of several prominent persons, including the poets Robert Burns and the romantic Lord
Byron, had been diagnosed as being due to this cause.

Indeed it has often been thought that this disease has a
special predilection for people of artistic temperament,
and in this connection we may recall that as a youth, the
poet, Alexander Pope, developed febrile attacks accompanied with severe shifting joint pains which recurred
throughout life. We read in a letter written two years
before his death, for instance, that: "Ever since I returned
home I have been in roaring pain, with a violent rheumatism in my left shoulder."

Again, the musical prodigy, Wolfgang Mozart, was taken at the age of six by his father to Vienna to entertain the Imperial Court. Sore throat, fever and pain, and swelling in his joints prevented his performance, however. Two days later he developed erythema nodosum of his shins and forearms. Such attacks recurred on many further occasions.

Subcutaneous nodules. Dr. William Charles Wells (1757–1817) was a colonial American subject who was compelled to leave his country during the War of Independence on account of his Royalist sympathies. A brilliant clinician, he was soon elected to the consulting staff of St. Thomas' Hospital in London, and to the Fellowship of the Royal Society. In 1812 he wrote his paper, *Rheumatism of the Heart*, in which we find the first mention of subcutaneous nodules in relation to rheumatism. He noted in a girl of fifteen, in hospital with acute rheumatism, that "many tendons of the superficial muscles of this patient were studded with numerous small hard tumours, an appearance I have observed in only one other person, who also laboured under rheumatism." He went on to say, however, that "they are probably much more frequently to be found than I myself have seen them. The same symptoms may have existed in several of my patients besides those of whom I have spoken." No further reference is to be found to rheumatic nodules for fifty years, when another American, Thomas Hillier, to whom original credit is often wrongly given, again described them in 1868.

In 1874 the French physician, Meynet, also wrote of them and rightly assessed their prognostic importance; they are often referred to in that country as "les nodes du Meynet" to this day. The most authoritative account, however, was finally given by Sir Thomas Barlow and Dr.

Francis Warner at the International Congress of Medicine in London in 1881. This was based upon twenty-seven cases observed by them over six years, and their conclusion was: "That in regard to the prognosis and treatment of the disease, although the nodules are unimportant in themselves, they are nevertheless of serious import, because in several cases the associated heart disease has been found actively progressive."

In 1819 Laennec announced his invention of the stethoscope, and with the help of this instrument the study of cardiac rheumatism progressed rapidly. Sir Charles Scudamore, in his *Treatise on the Nature and Cure of Gout*, mentioned in his edition of 1819 and in that of 1827, that he was impressed by "the remarkable predilection of the disease for synovial membranes, including the pericardium, endocardium and the dura mater." Of this he says further: "There is not probably a more dangerous form of disease than a sudden seizure of the pericardium during the inflammatory state of the system in acute rheumatism," a point which had first been put in evidence by William Balfour of Edinburgh in his *Observations* (1816).

James Hope (1801–1841), physician to St. George's Hospital, who died of tuberculosis at the zenith of a brilliant career, published a valuable *Treatise on the Diseases of the Heart and Great Vessels* (1832), in which he described individual valvular lesions as well as many disorders of cardiac rhythm; but as yet no one had recognised the most important lesion of all—myocarditis. Philippe Pinel (1745–1826), however, came close to anticipating Bouillaud's later work when commenting upon acute rheumatism's predilection for the muscular tissues, he said (1802) of the heart: "Enfin sa nature proprement musculaire l'expose-t'elle aux inflammations rhumatismales? Et par quels indices pourrait-on le reconnaître?"

The fourth period

Our fourth period begins with the publication by Jean-Baptiste Bouillaud (1796–1881), physician to the Sick Children's Hospital in Paris, of his great treatise *Nouvelles Recherches sur le Rhumatisme Articulaire* (1836). This starts in a low key: "On a first view of the subject it would seem that nothing could be more uninteresting or, one might say more played out, than a detailed treatise on rheumatism," but, he continues: "It is not so, however, and I venture to hope that the researches which constitute the body of this work will in fact offer some novelty and interest." With the help of his stethoscope and a great measure of clinical acumen, he was able to recognise and describe as a complete clinical and pathological entity for the first time rheumatic pancarditis. He also was able to offer a truer assessment of the injuries which this disease can inflict upon the heart. As he tersely put it: "Rheumatism licks the joints, the pleura and meninges, but bites the heart." He demonstrated that rheumatic pericarditis and endocarditis occur very frequently "and almost always accompany each other . . . and may in some measure be regarded as one of the elements of the disease." This obviously constituted a new conception of acute rheumatism. Rheumatic carditis could no longer be considered merely as an interesting complication of the disease, but as its most important manifestation. It was in formulating these ideas that Bouillaud's glory lies; and the attachment of his name to this disease in his own country seems justified.

Somewhat later he enunciated his famous "Law of

Coincidence" in which he embodied these truths: "In the great majority of cases of diffuse acute articular rheumatism with fever there exists in a variable degree a rheumatism of the serous-fibrous tissue of the heart. The coincidence is the rule, and non-coincidence the exception." On Bouillaud's work rests our modern conception of rheumatic fever and rheumatic carditis. It is curious that for the treatment of the condition this great physician should have continued to advocate savage bleeding, "coup sur coup," until the end of his life.

By 1843 Sir Thomas Watson, the President of the Royal College of Physicians and physician to the Middlesex Hospital, in his popular textbook, *Lectures on the Principles and Practice of Physic,* was able to discuss all aspects of acute rheumatism from a modern angle. He recognised well the increasing danger to the heart of recurrent attacks, and as a corollary the importance of rest as a treatment. When asked once by a student what was the best treatment for an attack of acute rheumatism he is said merely to have replied: "Six weeks!" His so-called law states: "The connection between the cardiac and the arthritic symptoms may be stated with confidence, namely, that the younger the patient is who suffers acute rheumatism, (and I have seen it as early as the third and fourth year), the more likely will he be to have rheumatic carditis. The chance of this combination appears to diminish after puberty, as life advances."

His colleague, Dr. Peter Mere Latham, also made prominent contributions to the fast-growing literature of this subject. He established the important point in his lectures to the students at St. Bartholomew's Hospital (1845), that:

> Cardiac manifestations are not more to be looked for when the disease is severe than when it is mild. Never omit,

therefore, to listen to the precordial region regularly whenever you visit a case of acute rheumatism—oftener perhaps
than you otherwise would do, merely for the sake of so
listening. All may seem to be going well. The general symptoms may seem far from severe. The chest may be free from
pain. The heart action may not awaken suspicion by its
force or irregularity. Nevertheless, its internal lining may be
inflamed, and if you listen, the endocardial murmur may
confirm the momentous fact directly to your ear.

He also did much to establish the importance of lung
involvement in acute rheumatism, a matter which continued to engage much serious attention of physicians
until recently.

About that time a curiously mediaeval theory was elaborated whereby the aetiology of the disease was attributed
to involvement of the central nervous system. To sustain
this view hypothetical centres for the control of joint
function, temperature regulation, and other reactions
were postulated as existing within the medulla oblongata.
This pseudo-physiological approach attracted considerable support for a time, even including that of Sir Jonathan Hutchinson and J. K. Mitchell.

Soon after this H. W. Fuller, in his book *On Rheumatism, Rheumatic Gout and Sciatica* (1852), put forward
the short-lived but much publicised theory that rheumatism and gout, although completely unconnected, were
in both cases a disease of abnormal metabolism. He suggested that lactic acid bears the same relationship to rheumatism that uric acid does to gout, and is in excess in
the blood. This theory was supported by Bouchard in
France, who initiated the "alkaline treatment," which by
means of various combinations of citrate and bicarbonate
salts administered frequently and in large doses should
aim to "restore the system to that alkaline condition which
is its due."

A further reactionary period supervened briefly, during which opinion reverted to the ancient conception of acute rheumatism and gout as clinical variants of the same underlying cause. The most vociferous exponents of this view, that a disturbance of the uric acid metabolism of the body was at fault, were P. W. Latham—in his Croonian lecture of 1886—and Dr. Alexander Haig (1853–1924), who wrote prolifically and lucratively along these lines. Haig pointed out, however, that whatever rheumatic poison was present in the system, it would require also a disturbing circumstance such as over-fatigue or anxiety as its exciting cause. This theory was finally discarded once more, however, for lack of any convincing confirmation. The whole situation was well summed up by the future Poet Laureate, Dr. Robert Bridges, when he wrote (1876): "Unfortunately the remedies which have through the ages been tried bear witness by their number to their inefficiency."

Pathology. The first serious histological investigation of the heart muscle in acute rheumatism was carried out by Dr. Samuel West, the founder of Great Ormond Street Children's Hospital, in 1878. He was able to confirm, after post-mortem examination, the presence of myocarditis in the case of a twenty-four-year-old woman in whom he had postulated this lesion during life. He reported "changes in the muscular wall of the ventricles which on microscopical examination proved to be areas that had undergone acute granular [fatty] degeneration." In 1889 appeared the classic work entitled *The Various Manifestations of the Rheumatic State as Exemplified in Childhood and Early Life,* by Dr. Walter B. Cheadle of St. Mary's Hospital. He consolidated the wider view of the disease, saying that "in the rheumatism of early life arthritis is at its minimum; endocarditis, pericarditis, chorea and subcutaneous nodules at their maximum."

Then follows a puzzling lack of further interest in the pathological aspects, except for the description of some microscopical interstitial lesions of which he did not apparently appreciate the importance, by F. J. Poynton, a pupil of Cheadle, in 1899; until 1904, when Karl Aschoff (1866–1942), then Professor of Pathology in the German University of Freiburg, published his famous work establishing the specific appearance and nature of those small interstitial lesions characteristic of rheumatic myocarditis which now bear his name, the "Aschoff nodes," or bodies. These constitute the counterpart in cardiac muscle of the subcutaneous fibrous nodule. He also pointed out rather later, with his assistant, Tawara (1906), that these submiliary nodules in the heart muscle could sometimes interfere with its conducting mechanism and so cause irregularities in rhythm, and even heart block. The invention of the electrocardiograph by Willem Einthoven about this time luckily enabled this aspect of pathology to be studied very fully. This laid the foundation for the modern specialty of cardiology which now flourishes in every civilised country.

The new science of bacteriology then initiated an active period of investigation which at first seemed to meet with little success. In 1900 Dr. F. J. Poynton, and Dr. A. Paine, announced their discovery of a small diplococcus in the blood and joint fluid of eight living children with acute rheumatism. This they proposed should be named the "Diplococcus rheumaticus." Subsequent investigations failed to substantiate the importance of this organism, however. As the result of later work the causative factor is today generally agreed to be a complicated reaction initiated by a Group A haemolytic streptococcus, which determines the immunological mechanisms causing the disease, as well as subsequent recurrences.

Treatment. One of the questions set by Professor John Eliotson in the first written examination ever held by the University of London (1833) was: "What are the chief remedies of rheumatism; the circumstances indicating the use of each; and the mode of employing each?" When we come to consider the answer to this it could largely be summarised in the words of P. M. Latham (1845), who said: "Acute rheumatism has experienced strange things at the hands of medical men. No disease has been treated by such various and opposite methods. Venesection and opium have wrought their cures, so has calomel. And so has colchicum, and so have drastic purgatives." Baillou had written that: "If pain and swelling of the joints remain after the fever is abated by means of frequent bleedings, apply 3 to 4 leeches to the parts, and let the blood ooze until it stops of itself." Bleeding remained the mainstay until the middle of the nineteenth century, in view of Bouillaud's reactionary advocacy of this age-long approach to the elimination of the causative "peccant humour." This was in spite of the words of his admired Sydenham, who had written of its treatment: "I judged it might be as successfully cured by a plain cooling and moderately nourishing diet as by repeated bleeding . . . and in reality it is much more serviceable than this [bleeding] and all the pompous garlands of drugs with which such who are willing to expire are crowned—as if they were beasts to be sacrificed."

Once the importance of cardiac involvement had been understood in the nineteenth century, rest was strongly advocated by Sir Thomas Watson and others. The phase during which alkaline treatment became popular followed and was based upon the belief that chill could inhibit the normal working of the sweat glands in the skin. These would, therefore, be unable to excrete lactic acid, which would accumulate in the bloodstream and so cause the manifestations of acute rheumatism. An "acid-free diet" designed to combat this disorder was devised by Alexander Haig and was for a time very fashionable.

Medicinally the Peruvian bark (quinine) had been, from Sydenham's time, the favourite drug; but therapeutic scepticism existed in academic circles, although its antipyretic action was recognised. Dr. Thomas MacLagan of Glasgow, like Haygarth at the opening of the century, erroneously believed acute rheumatism to be akin to malaria in nature: the result of a minute parasitic organism which lived in the marshy country where the disease flourished best (1876). The diseases being similar he thought that "there might—nay, there ought—to be some drug capable of exercising over its course the same controlling influence that quinine exercises over the course of ague." Being a very devout man and believing that God had arranged that natural remedies often lie not far from their causes, he sought some plant which also flourished in the same sort of countryside, and noticed the willow. He therefore tried the effect of salicin, the glucoside which had been extracted from its bark by Piria in 1839, and after first trying its effects upon himself, found it to be successful. Unfortunately, however, it was very expensive, the natural finished product costing twelve guineas per pound.

Unknown to him this effect of salicin had been discovered in similar fashion an hundred years previously by the Reverend Edmund Stone who reported to the Earl of Macclesfield, President of the Royal Society, on 25

April 1763, that: "Among the many useful discoveries there are very few which better deserve the attention of the Public than willow-bark. . . . About six years ago I accidentally tasted it and was surprised by its extraordinary bitterness, which raised the suspicion of its having the properties of Peruvian bark. As this tree delights in a moist and wet soil where agues abound, the general maxim that natural maladies carry their cures with them . . . was so very appropriate that I could not help applying it; and that this might be the intention of Providence I must own had some little weight with me." He tried it on about fifty sufferers with rheumatic fever during a period of five years, and he reported that it practically never failed. This work did not, however, become generally known.

In 1876 MacLagan published his results, and the specific action of the salicylate group of drugs in this disorder was thus soon widely established. Sodium salicylate, which had recently been synthesised by allowing carbon dioxide to act upon carbolic acid in the presence of an alkali (1874), was now on the market and being less toxic was soon substituted for salicin at the suggestion of the German Professor Hermann Senator. Later still, from 1899 onwards, sodium acetylsalicylate (aspirin) became generally adopted, being in tablet form easier to take, of less unpleasant taste, and causing less gastric irritation; whilst its price was now only twelve shillings a pound.

During the second and third decades of the present century it became customary to administer salicylates in conjunction with large doses of sodium bicarbonate, as it was found that they could be more easily tolerated and side effects did not occur. After the introduction of plasma-level estimations, however, it was soon noted by Dr. Coburn of Baltimore, that alkalis greatly increased the rate of excretion of the salicylates, so that in this way most of it was ineffective, not reaching the affected tissues.

In 1949, after the discovery of the therapeutic anti-inflammatory effect of the steroid hormones by Philip Hench and E. C. Kendall, which won them the Nobel Prize, it was thought that these drugs might substitute for the salicylates. It is now generally considered, however, that since both groups can be seen satisfactorily to control the exudative phenomena of acute rheumatism, nothing is normally gained by such substitution.

Cardiac Surgery. Sir Henry Souttar was the first surgeon purposefully to open the living human heart. He operated at the London Hospital in 1925 on a girl of sixteen suffering with mitral stenosis and regurgitation and attempted to stretch the contracted valve. For various reasons no further development occurred, however, in this sphere until Sir Russell Brock in London and Professor Alfred Blalock at Johns Hopkins more recently succeeded in establishing cardiac surgery as a safe and helpful procedure.

The advent of methods of inducing hypothermia and the development of machines permitting of extra-corporeal circulation of the bloodstream are leading to continued expansion in this branch of surgery.

In the preventive field the chief advance which has taken place during the last twenty years is the so-called "interval treatment" with sulphonamides, or with antibiotics such as penicillin. The intention is to prevent re-infection with the haemolytic streptococci which are now known to be the determining cause of recurrent attacks. In this way the grave danger of development of severe heart disease has been greatly reduced.

The other main advance has lain in the provision of help for the sufferers with disabling heart disease, together with the promotion of further research, by social organisations and government authorities. As Sir John Parkinson has recently said: "The recent history of acute rheumatism centres mostly on the realisation that it is not only a large professional problem, but also one of vital public and national interest concerning children." This viewpoint started in England in 1888, when the British Medical Association organised the first collective investigation into the disease, covering not only its clinical features but also the influence of social factors, habits, and locality. This formed the basis for the well-known *Report to the Local Government Body* by Sir Arthur Newsholme (1895), which inaugurated government interest in the subject. This was soon followed in the United States and later in most other civilised countries, by further social surveys and appropriate legislative and other action.

Finale

So we have followed through its vicissitudes a disease which at the outset of our story was considered merely as an articular throw-back from the important group of gouty disorders. This gradually assumed a position which has achieved for it the status of a special department in the World Health Organisation. It is appropriate to end with Poynton's final assessment in 1936 of the status of rheumatic fever, which is still true, namely:

> It is a chronic systemic infection subject to intervals of apparent recovery alternating with periods of activity affecting chiefly the cardiovascular system, particularly the heart, and possessing a marked tendency to affect the human organism before puberty. Its manifestations are numerous, and it is apparent now that the seemingly insignificant "growing-pains" of which many young children complain are as highly rheumatic and as full of possible danger to health and life as a severe attack of polyarthritis.

It constitutes the delayed result of a sometimes trivial throat infection with a special type of haemolytic streptococcus; and today most authorities have come to the conclusion that there is probably also a genetic factor to be reckoned with in most cases. No doubt some way will be found in due course whereby the relative importance of the various factors concerned may be assessed in every individual patient, and the disease altogether prevented.

Chorea, or St. Vitus' Dance

Chorea, which is now regarded as a curious variant of acute rheumatism, was first described by Thomas Sydenham, after whom it is often named "Sydenham's chorea." St. Vitus, a Roman missionary who was boiled in oil by the ungrateful citizens of Ulm in A.D. 303, was the reputed patron of "Rock an' Roll" through the ages. Sufferers with all forms of "the dancing malady" could be cured by a visit to his shrine. Thus he became associated with this disorder in the popular mind. Sydenham did not himself connect the disease in any way with the field of rheumatism. His account is to be found in his last work, *Schedula monitoria* (1686):

> Chorea of St. Vitus. This disorder is a kind of convulsion which seizes children of both sexes from the tenth to the fourteenth year; it manifests itself by a halting or misteadiness of one of the legs which the patient draws after him like an idiot. If the hand of the same side be applied to the breast, or any other part of the body, the child cannot keep it there a moment in the same posture, but it will be drawn into a different one by a convulsion, notwithstanding all his efforts to the contrary. Before the child who hath this disorder can get a glass or cup to his mouth he useth abundance of odd gestures; for he does not bring it in a straight line thereto, but his hand being drawn sideways by

the spasm he moves it backwards and forwards till at length
the glass accidentally coming nearer his lips he throws the
liquor hastily into his mouth and swallows it greedily, as if
he meant to divert the spectators.

Sydenham thought that small doses of laudanum were of
help in calming the paroxysms of this malady.

There seems to have been no further mention of this
condition until Sir Charles Scudamore's *Treatise on the
Nature and Cure of Gout* (1816) in which he says that he
had occasionally seen chorea following acute rheumatism,
although he was inclined to think that in such cases the
rheumatism might only be acting in the role of a predisposing agent, preparing the soil for a nervous manifestation.

Three years later Dr. B. G. Babington, physician to
Guy's Hospital, pointed out for the first time the frequency with which a mitral murmur might be heard in
the course of an attack of chorea, by the use of that recently introduced instrument, the stethoscope. His actual
words are of considerable interest and may be quoted
from the *Guy's Hospital Reports* (1821): "Out of a large
number of cases of chorea seen lately by my friend and
colleague, Dr. Addison, to whom I am indebted for first
having directed my attention to this point, only two
have been without a decided mitral or left ventricular
bruit." Following this line of investigation he eventually
came to the conclusion that chorea must be due to a
lesion of the heart, for he said: "Should further investigation prove chorea to be more immediately dependent
upon disease of the heart or pericardium than has been
hitherto supposed, the merit of this discovery will certainly be due to Dr. Addison." This reference is naturally
to Dr. Thomas Addison, who later was to describe that

form of anaemia and the disease of the adrenal bodies, both of which still bear his name.

Their distinguished colleague, Dr. Richard Bright, also lent the weight of his great authority to this thesis. In his Lumleian lecture before the Royal College of Physicians in 1837 he said: "The great and important point is . . . the fact that the most violent attacks of this spasmodic disease will occasionally owe their existence to inflammation of that portion of pleura and pericardium."

We begin to approach the modern view with the report by Dr. James Begbie in the *Monthly Journal of Medical Science* (1847), of a rheumatic family of four individuals, two of whom were suffering with acute articular rheumatism of the usual painful type, one with the typical chorea, and one less fortunate still was suffering with both conditions—a combination that Mark Twain thought might well prove a suitable fate to be accorded to the damned. From a close study of this family and other cases Begbie decided that: "The same diathesis which under certain circumstances leads to the production of the one [rheumatism], in different conditions tends to the development of the other [chorea]." He reasoned, correctly, therefore that the two syndromes were independent of each other although born of the same underlying cause.

J. P. Botral, in his thesis for the Doctorate of the University of Paris in 1850, was still a little more explicit in saying that "Chorea, it seems to me, should be considered at this time as a rheumatic infection [*sic*], and as having as its physiological basis a rheumatism of the central nervous system."

Numerous theories continued to be advanced, however, to substantiate the cardiac origin of chorea, and as late as 1890 we find Sir Archibald Garrod stating in his *Treatise*

on Rheumatism and Rheumatoid Arthritis that: "Physicians whose opinions are entitled to the greatest respect
have held, and still hold, that endocarditis in chorea is
either due to chorea itself, or is a result of mental shock
which so often precedes its onset; or that both chorea and
the endocarditis are manifestations of some morbid
process allied to, but not identical with, rheumatism."

Drs. F. J. Poynton and A. Paine of Great Ormond
Street Children's Hospital reported in 1901 that they
believed that they had proved, both microscopically and
experimentally, that chorea was a rheumatic meningo-
encephalitis. They described correctly the evidence of
diffuse congestion which affects all parts, and the degenerative changes seen in the nerve cells; but the organism
which they described as causative has not withstood the
test of time.

The treatment advocated by Poynton was modern. He
emphasised the importance of procuring for the child
prolonged mental as well as physical rest, and in pursuance of this often incurred the wrath of parents and
visitors by excluding them from his ward until the patient
was convalescent. He would also exert his authority
against sending them for convalescence at the seaside,
for he thought that the restlessness of the waves produced
an undesirable and similar effect on the type of child who
tended to be liable to this affliction. Medicinally he
would prescribe aspirin in large doses to reduce the
tendency to rheumatic carditis; sedatives for the period
during which they were required; and an ample and
nutritious diet, supplemented with cod-liver oil. He
opposed the contemporary view that arsenic in large
dosage should be prescribed in these cases. He believed
that if this had any effect it was to produce a peripheral

neuritis—a wrong way in which to seek to calm the patient's unwanted movements.

This disease is seen less frequently nowadays, but its treatment remains much the same as it was in Dr. Poynton's time, and the results are similar. It is usual now to give lessons in hospital as divertional therapy because failure to keep up with their school contemporaries can cause psychological difficulties later. "Play-therapy" is also generally added, to regain muscle co-ordination of the finer movements and to restore the child's self-confidence. Recurrence, once remission has been established, is now a very rare event.

CHAPTER IX

Rheumatoid Arthritis

Until comparatively recently medical writers were unable to draw much distinction between the different types of chronic arthritis. Early observers considered them all to be variants of gout, although later it was recognised that this was not necessarily so; and during the seventeenth century the terms "scorbutic arthritis" and "rheumatism" were coined as useful verbal rubbish heaps to which all non-gouty arthritis could be consigned.

There seems to be no doubt, however, that although it only received its name just over a hundred years ago, rheumatoid arthritis is a disease with a long pedigree. Sir Grafton Elliot Smith, for example, disinterred many prehistoric skeletons in Egypt, in which traces of this disease could be recognised. His colleague, Frederick Wood-Jones, is quoted by J. D. Comrie as claiming that chronic arthritis was the bone disease *par excellence* of the ancient Nubians as almost every skeleton he examined showed signs, often severe, of its ravages. Many of the bones which were uncovered when the site of Pompeii was first excavated were examined by Charcot, who reported (1862) that many of them clearly demonstrated similar lesions.

It seems quite likely that Hippocrates was describing cases of rheumatoid arthritis when he wrote:

> In the arthritis which generally shows itself about the age of thirty-five there is frequently no great interval between the affection of the hands and the feet; both these becoming similar in nature, slender, with little flesh. Their tempera-

ture approximates to the external cold, far from the body's heat. For the most part their arthritis passeth from the feet to the hands, next the elbows and the knees, after these the hip joint. It is incredible how far the mischief spreads.

That distinguished Byzantine-Greek physician, Soranus of Ephesus, writing during the second century A.D., may also have had it in mind when he wrote, in his treatise *On Acute and Chronic Diseases,* that the distinction between chronic arthritis and chronic podagra:

> is, of course, very clear and obvious, for podagra is a disease only of the feet, whilst chronic arthritis is a disease of all the joints, or several of them. The arthritis sometimes begins at the feet and later involves the other joints; whilst sometimes it begins in the joints themselves and later involves the feet. Thus some physicians call arthritis the general class, and podagra a species of the class. . . . Arthritis cannot simply be identified with podagra . . . but in a discussion of treatments we need not argue about these things . . . as clearly they are all of the same general type.

He also mentioned that arthritis, unlike podagra, is common in women, and even eunuchs and children, as well as middle-aged men. He noticed that its onset was often determined by some sudden unaccustomed physical or mental stress; and also sometimes when physically active life was deserted for one of sloth and luxury. He made special reference to that curse of the rheumatoid sufferer, morning stiffness.

Scribonius Largus, who accompanied Julius Caesar as his chief medical officer on his successful invasion of Britain and returned to prosperous practice in Rome, also wrote, but in less specific terms, of "that chronic polyarthritis which occurs chiefly in elderly women."

Infective Forms

Infective arthritis of various sorts was confused with rheumatoid polyarthritis until quite recently. Soranus, in describing the hot and cold varieties of chronic arthritis, may unknowingly have been making this distinction. The older Greek physicians were also aware that arthritis might follow "fevers."

Gonorrhoea

It was Dr. William Musgrave of Exeter (1657–1721), the later Secretary of the Royal Society, who first drew attention to the occurrence of polyarthritis as a sequel to gonorrhoea. This was confirmed in 1786 by John Hunter in his book on the venereal diseases although he added that he had never seen syphilis attack the joints. It is less obvious what value to put on Hunter's further statements that:

> Rheumatism in many of its symptoms and in some consti-tutions resembles the *lues venerea* . . . thus many rheu-matic complaints are cured by mercury and thereafter are supposed to have been of venereal origin. Mercury given without caution often produces the same symptoms as rheumatism, and I have, for this reason, even seen in such cases this medicine continued.

He clearly recognised that the movement of infected joints of this type would lead to deformities: "Nothing can promote contracture of a joint so much as motion before the disease is removed." He rightly went on to say, how-ever, that: "When all inflammation is gone off a little motion frequently repeated is necessary."

Sir Benjamin Brodie, of St. George's Hospital, gave a masterly description of a case of arthritis of gonococcal causation in his pioneer book *Observations on Dis-*

eases of the Joints (1818). He also delineated a case of what is now called Reiter's disease in a man of forty-five, of which he said: "The following case furnishes an example of a disease which as far as I know has not been described by any pathological or surgical writer previously." This was almost exactly two hundred years prior to Reiter's own description. In 1879 final full confirmation of the gonococcal variety of arthritis was achieved by Albert Neisser, who described his finding of the causative organism in the joint fluid aspirated from such a case, the *gonococcus* which bears his name.

Tuberculosis

Tuberculous infection of joints is thought to have been common amongst the ancient, as amongst the modern, Greeks. Although not recognised as being basically different from other forms of arthritis until the discovery of the tuberculosis bacillus by Robert Koch in 1882, certain writers described cases which appear to have been of this nature. Hippocrates mentions arthritis in which the muscles surrounding the affected joint waste away, leaving it swollen and unsupported; and mentions that such patients usually die. Soranus described the "cold variety" of joint swelling; and much later Musgrave described the *tumor albus,* or white swelling, which he rightly associated with a "scrofulous diathesis." In 1909 Professor Poncet of Lyons postulated that certain cases of generalised rheumatoid arthritis were due to a blood-borne tuberculous infection. This he named "tuberculous rheumatism," but the existence of such a syndrome has never finally been established. A similar, equally unproved concept, was advanced in favour of syphilis as the cause of a chronic progressive polyarthritis.

Not much further attention was paid to the infective

category of arthritis until after the birth of general bacteriology, when Strangeways, in 1905, confirmed the observations which Heberden (1802) and Bouchard (1891) had recorded, namely that polyarthritis of rheumatoid type can result from infection following diseases as diverse as scarlet fever, pneumonia, dysentery (flux), and Malta fever (brucellosis).

Baillou had written (1642) that: "Rheumatism must be regarded as the prodromal sign and predisposing cause of arthritis," by which he meant that the cause of rheumatoid arthritis is rheumatic fever, a belief which is still occasionally held. Sydenham, by the seventeenth century, had realised that there were categories of arthritis which lay outside those two syndromes of gout and acute rheumatism which he so clearly differentiated for the first time. These other types he designated "scorbutic rheumatisms," which he intended as a generic term; but amongst these we can discern the outlines of rheumatoid arthritis. As a devout believer in the humoral hypothesis, whereby the pathology of all diseases is the result of changes in the four circulating humours, however, the possibility of various forms having different aetiologies would scarcely have occurred to him.

In 1763 Sauvages described a secondary type of rheumatic joint disease which may follow sudden chilling or trauma. He said that it might produce swellings of the finger joints "about the size and shape of an hazel nut, (rhumatisme noyeux), but never concretions such as occur in the gout. . . . It is not periodic in its attacks like the rheumatism, but frequently presents mild paroxysms which involve the hands, the feet and the knees. The fingers and hands become deformed and twisted; and it lasts until death." This seems a recognisable picture of rheumatoid arthritis. Luckily, posterity neglected the fifteen further varieties into which he proposed to classify arthritis. William Heberden also, in his *Commentaries* (1802), described the chronic types of rheumatism, mentioning the great deterioration in general health which is observed to accompany this form, as well as the local effects of the contractures of joints and muscles which commonly occur.

Cullen prefaced his observations (1763) by saying: "Rheumatism—this is a common subject, but however common, like most other subjects in physic it admits of a great deal of discussion." He surveyed the field fully and also made the original statement that a chronic form of rheumatism will sometimes be produced if too much blood is removed during the treatment of acute rheumatism or gout by this method. As an example of what he was condemning he said: "I have known in this country both arms set a-bleeding at once a twelve ounces or even one pound of blood taken from each." More frequently, however, he thought that chronic arthritis was caused by the sudden chilling of joints which had become congested, and that it was for this reason that such diseases occurred more commonly during the cold winter months, "arthritis a frigore." The phenomenon of reflex muscular wasting was observed by John Hunter who reported (1776) that: "The lesions that involve the ligaments, the tendons . . . disturb the functions of the muscles to a greater degree than those that involve the muscles themselves, in that such lesions, by sympathy, cause atrophy."

It was only with the dawning of the nineteenth century that the type of polyarthritis which we now term rheumatoid arthritis became clearly differentiated. In 1805 John Haygarth of Bath described a chronic arthritis starting in the finger joints and progressing until most of the other joints were affected, with much distortion. He was impressed by the determining role of the menopause in a large number of his cases. He remarked gloomily that: "This is a disease which sadly embitters, but does not shorten, the duration of life"; and named it "nodosity of the joints," saying: "In giving it this distinct name I hope that it may henceforward be considered as a separate genus, and become a more special object of medical enquiry." Robert Adams, whilst agreeing, pointed out that the property of hardness which the term "nodosity" suggested was inappropriate, as "the swellings of the joints which we notice in this disease are by no means hard; on the contrary, as in its early stages the swellings are principally constituted by the effusion of much synovial fluid into the interior of the joints, they are soft and fluctuating."

It was a young French doctor, Augustin Landré-Beauvais, who later became physician to the Salpêtrière Hospital in Paris, who in 1800 gave the description of the disease to which priority is generally accorded, in his thesis for the M.D. This he presented under the title of *La Goutte Asthénique Primitive des Jointures*. He noted that thirty-three of his thirty-four cases were women, and described its most striking features. He stated: "There is a painful and troublesome disease of the joints of a peculiar nature. It is clearly distinguishable from all others by symptoms manifestly different from the gout, and from acute and chronic rheumatism."

Sir Charles Scudamore (1779–1849) wrote the first work to be devoted to the study of the rheumatic diseases as a group, *A Treatise on the Nature and Cure of Gout*, which appeared in 1816, dedicated to Matthew Baillie, John Hunter's nephew. This was based upon his own observation of about one hundred patients whom he kept under review; but few of these appear to have been of rheumatoid type. A second edition was called for in 1817, followed by several others at further short intervals. In 1853 Charcot published his doctoral thesis on the disease known variously as "Goutte Asthénique Primitive," "Nodosités des Jointures," and "Rhumatisme Articulaire Chronique," in which he gave a good clinical description of rheumatoid arthritis illustrated with a series of his own remarkable drawings of the contractures of the joints.

H. W. Fuller of St. George's Hospital, in his book *On Rheumatism, Rheumatic Gout and Sciatica* (1854) also gave a good description of rheumatoid arthritis, calling it rheumatic gout, but emphasising that it had no real affinity with gout. It was the distinguished Dublin physician and anatomist, Robert Adams, however, who first succeeded in interesting the British medical profession as a whole in rheumatoid arthritis, under the name of "chronic rheumatic arthritis," by the publication in London of his fine *Treatise on the Rheumatic Gout, or Chronic Rheumatic Arthritis of All the Joints* (1857). As he pointed out in the preface, he had had exceptionally favourable opportunities for studying the disease in all its stages, as it was exceedingly common amongst the poor in Ireland—indeed he proposed at one time to name it "arthritis pauperum"; and since the death rate from other causes was high it was not difficult to obtain affected joints for post-mortem study. He established it as a constitutional disease affecting many joints simultaneously, describing morning stiffness as a characteristic feature, and pointing out its inflammatory basis. He thought true bony ankylosis to be rare, and referred to the possibility of spontaneous clinical remission, even when the disease had lasted many years.

Sir Alfred Garrod's distinctive separation of gout from

other forms of arthritis, by his discovery of an excess of uric acid in the blood of patients suffering with the former disease, enabled rheumatoid arthritis to be differentiated clearly, and named by him, in his book *Gout and Rheumatic Gout* (1859), which he wrote whilst assistant physician to the West London Hospital. His actual words may be quoted once again:

> The term "rheumatic gout" is given particularly by the medical profession, to a disease having a peculiar pathology in no way related to gout, and not necessarily to rheumatism. . . . Although unwilling to add to the number of names, I cannot help expressing a desire that one might be found for this disease, not implying any necessary relation between it and either gout or rheumatism. Perhaps *Rheumatoid Arthritis* would answer the object; by which term I should wish to imply an inflammatory condition of the joints not unlike rheumatism in some of its characters, but differing materially from it.

Variants

In 1897 Sir George Frederick Still, whilst he was still a resident at the Great Ormond Street Children's Hospital, London, described a juvenile form of rheumatoid arthritis in which the spleen and the lymphatic glands were generally enlarged. Very shortly afterwards the French physician, Anatole Chauffard, independently published a description of this syndrome, which is accordingly often known eponymously as the Chauffard-Still disease.

An adult variant of rheumatoid arthritis, in which the lymphatic glands and the spleen are also enlarged and the white cells of the blood diminished, was described in five cases seen at the Johns Hopkins Hospital in 1924 by A. R. Felty, whose name has subsequently been attached to this syndrome. The association of rheumatoid arthritis with other disease processes, such as ulcerative colitis, and the skin lesions of psoriasis has been remarked upon frequently, in the first instance, by that obsessional observer and great dermatologist Jean Louis Alibert in his *Maladies de la Peau* (1806). Pierre Bazin, another celebrated skin physician coined the name "arthropathica psoriatica" in 1860 to describe this syndrome.

Causes of Rheumatoid Arthritis

The death knell of humoral pathology was sounded by the publication of Morgagni's great work *Seats and Causes of Diseases Investigated by Anatomy* (1761), which was the first work to delineate morbid anatomy in detail. For the first time it showed that different diseases exhibit localised pathological changes peculiar to each.

So speculation regarding the specific aetiology of disease increased throughout the eighteenth century, as belief in the humoral hypothesis waned. Dr. William Oliver, a celebrated physician who served in the rebel Duke of Monmouth's army, and who was the founder of the rheumatic hospital at Bath, and who also invented a popular biscuit still sold as "the original Bath Oliver," wrote in 1751 of chronic arthritis that: " 'Tis certain a most stubborn distemper, and has baffled all the professors of Physick that ever have appeared in the World. The cause lies too deep for any Medicine or Method yet known to come to the bottom of it." Subsequent writers attributed it mostly to chill, trauma, or as the sequel to acute rheumatism or gout.

Towards the middle of the nineteenth century J. K. Mitchell of Philadelphia (the father of the more celebrated S. Weir Mitchell), Robert Remak of Berlin, and others, advanced the hypothesis that the joint changes in rheumatoid arthritis are due to primary changes occurring in the central nervous system—"arthritis myelitica." They based their view largely upon the bilateral and symmetrical distribution of the joint lesions commonly observed in its early stages; and on the selective muscular wasting which so often occurs in the hands and arms, and the well-attested fact that its onset may be determined by shock. For a time such European celebrities as Jean Charcot, Sir Jonathan Hutchinson, and Sir Alfred Garrod also subscribed to this view, although no anatomical confirmatory evidence was ever produced.

The microscopical appearances of the joint synovium were described by Garrod in 1848 as being inflammatory in nature. It was consequently assumed that such changes must result from some generalised infection, more particularly as polyarthritis had been known since the time of Hippocrates to follow certain fevers. Bacteriology was in its infancy and many workers approached the problem of rheumatoid arthritis from this aspect with enthusiasm. All, however, failed to find evidence which convinced of general infection.

In 1810 Benjamin Rush, a founder of the Pennsylvania General Hospital, who enjoyed the friendship of both Jefferson and Franklin, and was himself a signatory of the Declaration of Independence, had introduced, in his *Medical Enquiries and Observations,* the conception that dental sepsis might cause general disease, and described the cure of a case of arthritis as the result of removing an infected tooth. He said later: "I have been made happy by discovering that I have only added to the observations of other physicians in pointing out a connection between the extraction of decayed or diseased teeth and the cause and cure of disease,"—a modest statement, typical of one who was designated "the American Sydenham." This conception was elaborated and formalised in 1912 by F. Billings as "the hypothesis of Focal Sepsis," which held sway until recently.

Garrod's assertion that the changes in this disease were inflammatory in nature was challenged by Todd, as nothing, he pointed out, resembling pus was ever found in affected joints; he thought that "irritation would be a more correct term," and that this might originate in abnormal nutrition, resulting in the presence of "a peculiar matter" in the nutrient joint fluid. The ancient Greek physician, Aetius, had voiced a similar opinion when he said: "It neither comes to suppuration like other humours, nor for that as I think because it happens in bloodless parts, but through the occasion of some specific malignity."

In 1905 Dr. T. S. P. Strangeways, with a small personal legacy, bought two little houses in Cambridge for a hospital, and set up a laboratory in the coal shed, in order to study "rheumatoid arthritis and such other special diseases the pathology and treatment of which are as yet undetermined." With the rise of bacteriology he was able to confirm that polyarthritis of rheumatoid type can result from certain general infective processes such as scarlet fever, gonorrhoea, and dysentery, but could not show that the classical type resulted directly from infection. He concluded that further advances in this subject would have to be sought at the cellular level, and acting on this belief, he eventually pioneered the science and technique of tissue culture. As a result, the idea of focal sepsis from a hidden source of infection somewhere in the body was reinforced, largely by William Hunter (1901), Willcox, and others, and as antibiotics had not yet been discovered many teeth, tonsils, and antral linings, as well as symptomless gall bladders and appendices, doubtfully condemned, were subsequently sacrificed needlessly on the altar of this hypothesis, which as mentioned above, held the field *faut de mieux* until recent times. Thus medical opinion, until the third decade of our own century, had practically reverted to the humoral hypothesis of Galen by postulating a toxic substance of unknown origin, produced by a hypothetical "focus" somewhere in the body, and having a selective affinity for weakened joints.

Modern conceptions of aetiology may seem equally unprecise, but are more firmly based on scientific methods. In 1948 it was confirmed that a specific substance of unknown nature, similar to an antibody, and named the "rheumatoid factor," circulated in the blood of rheumatoid sufferers. It was on the detection of this factor that such modern diagnostic procedures as the Rose-Waaler and the Latex tests are based. A great volume of work has been carried out in the United States and in Great Britain during the last ten years to identify the nature and function of this rheumatoid factor; and the present trend seems to incriminate as the cause of rheumatoid arthritis a state of altered immunity or auto-immunity, probably with the addition of a genetic or metabolic predisposing factor. (It is interesting to recall that William Heberden mentioned, in the appendix to his *Commentaries*, that chronic arthritis will sometimes be hereditary.) The concept now generally held of rheumatoid arthritis as one of the group of connective-tissue diseases was enunciated by Klinge about twenty years ago. Indeed, the classification drawn up by the World Health Organisation (1956) confers upon the "collagen group" of diseases the synonymous title of "Para-Rheumatic Diseases."

Pathology

The first descriptive and illustrated account of the pathological changes observed in the joints in rheumatoid arthritis, as we have seen, was that of Robert Adams (1857). Others who wrote notably upon this subject were John Kent Spender of Bath, who also described the patches of skin pigmentation which may occur during the disease, which are often named after him "Spender's Spots." Jean Charcot published in Paris his celebrated *Clinical Lectures on Chronic Diseases* in 1881, in which he put back the pathological clock by decreeing that all forms of chronic arthritis, other than those due to gout, were merely variants and should all be described under the single heading "Rhumatisme articulaire chronique progressif." This view was also advanced by the German pathologist, Rudolf Virchow, who coined the term "arthritis deformans" to cover all forms of chronic arthritis. It was unfortunate that the material available to these two great men originated from their geriatric wards, and so led to this erroneous conclusion.

It was G. A. Bannatyne, a Scottish physician who practised in Bath, to whom credit should go for differentiating the pathological changes found in the joints of sufferers with active rheumatoid arthritis and osteoarthritis. This he did in the fourth edition of his book *Rheumatoid Arthritis, its Pathology, Morbid Anatomy and Treatment*, which was first published in 1896 and was the first medical book to show an X-ray illustration. He believed rheumatoid arthritis to be a generalised microbic disease, osteoarthritis the result of senile changes. This work was improved upon, notably by A. E. Garrod and such men as Strangeways and Lawford Knaggs. After the introduction of X-ray photography by Röntgen, Goldthwait of Boston produced a classification of arthritis (1904) based upon the differing radiological appearances of rheumatoid arthritis and osteoarthritis, and proposed the names "atrophic" and "hypertrophic" which are still occasionally employed. In 1915 Nichols and Richardson of the same city proposed a further classification and nomenclature based upon pathological findings, in which they proposed to name the two main types of arthritis "proliferative" and "degenerative." A committee investigating this matter between the wars reported that no fewer than sixty synonyms had by then been employed to designate arthritis of the type named by Garrod "rheumatoid." This term was finally adopted for use in the United States in 1941.

John Kent Spender also pointed out (1889) certain aetiological affinities which he believed to exist between the early phases of rheumatoid arthritis and cases of hyperthyroidism and certain other disease states, a matter which is again receiving attention, particularly in the field of immunology.

Sir Archibald Garrod (1857–1936), who was the fourth son of Sir Alfred, published *A Treatise on Rheumatism and Rheumatoid Arthritis* (1890). His avowed aim was to present a consistent picture of rheumatoid disease in all its manifestations as a generalised systemic disorder. He thought that the forms in which it was presented might be modified by environmental factors, but believed that they depended upon a specific morbid process. Although he later drew the historic distinction based on Bannatyne's work between the pathological appearances of rheumatoid arthritis and osteoarthritis for the first time (1907), he frequently appeared to confuse their clinical manifestations, and even refers to Heberden's nodes as "rheumatoid." He analysed the many notes on rheumatoid cases left by his father, and recorded *inter alia* that a family history could be traced in no less than 16.8 per cent; that of his first five hundred cases, 411 were women; and that he had established the existence of an acute mode of onset, differing from acute rheumatism. The list of favourite treatments for this disease which Sir Archibald said were current in his time is also of interest, and includes hyperpyrexia, hypothermia, shock therapy, subcutaneous injection of distilled water or carbon dioxide, ichthyol, formic acid, and other procedures now mostly forgotten.

Weather-Sensitivity

It has always been claimed by rheumatic sufferers, particularly those with rheumatoid arthritis, that they become endowed with the interesting faculty of predicting the weather and its changes. This claim is mentioned in the earliest-known English textbook of medicine, John of Gaddesden's *Rosa Anglica*. He said: "That variations in the weather can cause this malady one knows well; arthritics can predict bad weather, and at the outset of shower or storm they cannot rest at ease." The great French surgeon, Ambroise Paré, may have had this passage in mind when he wrote: "Gouty patients can feel and perceive changes in the weather such as rain, snow, winds and suchlike, as though they had within them built in an almanac to last their lifetime." This aspect has been reappraised scientifically during the last few years in the University of Pennsylvania. With the help of a "Climatron," a chamber in which rheumatoid patients lived under varying conditions of temperature, dampness, and barometric pressure, it was shown that when conditions were adjusted, unknown to the inmates, to simulate those of an approaching storm, they spontaneously complained of "feeling it in their bones."

Incidence

It is impossible to estimate the frequency of rheumatoid arthritis in the past, although it is probable in spite of its late recognition as a separate clinical entity, that it was common then as now. Of the sixty-five patients who were admitted to the new hospital of St. George's in London in 1734, five were recorded as suffering with "rheumatism," and one died. During the years 1775–1780 the admissions for chronic arthritis with muscle wasting amounted to 362. The *London Directory* (1818) guesses the incidence of "chronic rheumatisms" at 1:25 of the hospital population. The majority of these we may perhaps presume were rheumatoid sufferers. Haygarth (1805) gave the incidence as 1:310 of the population (0.32 per cent). In a recent population survey taken in England and Wales by the Empire Rheumatism Council, this disease was found to account for two to four per cent of all diseases applying for treatment. It was estimated in 1956 that there were four to six million sufferers with rheumatoid arthritis in the United States.

Celebrated Sufferers

The world nearly lost the services of one of its notable Popes, Pius II, owing to the fact that for several years prior to his election "he lay sick and ill between burning spasms of fever and pain," unable to undertake that last Crusade against the Turks, which was his life's ambition. His sufferings were diagnosed by his physician as due to gout, but perusal of his fascinating autobiography suggests that the disease was rheumatoid arthritis. When, after the stormily contested papal election, all the Cardinals fell at his feet and saluted him as Pope, the leader of the opposition excused himself for having voted against him, saying: "Your Holiness, we approve your election. We think you worthy of this great office. The reason we did not vote for you was your infirmity. We thought your arthritis the one thing against you, for the Church needs an active man. But since God is satisfied we must needs be satisfied too." He soon showed himself one of the most dynamic leaders of fifteenth-century Christendom.

It is difficult to pick out with certainty those other important figures in history who doubtless suffered with rheumatoid arthritis. It would seem probable, however, that Christopher Columbus (1451–1506) was a victim. It is recorded that whilst he was on his third crossing of the Atlantic, in the caravel, "Niña," in June, 1498: "After they had advanced within the tropics the change of climate brought on the gout of all his joints accompanied with a low fever." About the same time he suffered several severe and painful attacks of ophthalmia, which is not uncommonly a complication of rheumatoid arthritis. Two years later, after a period of great mental stress and anxiety—"nervous and overwrought with much worry"—all his joints are said to have become constantly swollen and aching, and he had to be roped to the mast in bad weather that he might not be swept overboard. In 1502 he started on his last voyage from Cadiz in poor general health. On his return from that disastrous venture his arthritis became permanent, and he found himself too crippled to obey his monarch's summons to Court that he might render an account of his exploits. He died in 1506 with great swelling of his legs and belly, possibly of heart failure.

Another well-documented sufferer is Mary, Queen of Scots (1542–1587), whose arthritic sufferings have been

chronicled by Sir Arthur MacNalty in his book of that
name (1961). The first mention of painful swelling of
her joints was during her imprisonment on Loch Leven
in 1566, which occurred after an acute exacerbation of a
gastric ulcer. Gradually her neck, hands, and elbows became involved and later we hear of her right arm being
badly crippled. Soon she had to be carried in a chair by
attendants: "not being allowed the command of my legs";
and during the next few years "she was so ill with pains
in her limbs that she could not turn in her bed." As
sometimes occurs in this disease, however, it suddenly
went into remission, and in the year before her death she
was again able to ride a horse and even go hunting.

During her custody by the Earl of Shrewsbury she
petitioned, on several occasions successfully, to be allowed to go for warm-bath treatment at the neighbouring
spa of Buxton, which he owned. This always gave her
great relief for a time. When the end came she was again
considerably crippled, and had to be supported on one
side by a lady-in-waiting and on the other by her physician, Bourgoing, to enable her to walk along the cor-
ridor from her room in Fotheringay Castle to the Great
Hall and ascend the scaffold which had been erected there
for her execution.

Her contemporary and judge, Archbishop Parker, also
recorded that in his latter years, owing to the rheumatic
swelling of all his joints, he was no longer able to cross
the Thames from his palace at Lambeth to attend meet-
ings of the Privy Council in Westminster. It may have
been on this account that he was not present at the
meeting at which it was decided that proceedings must
be taken against Dr. John Caius, the Master of Gonville
and Caius College, and some other members of his old
University who were suspected of favouring the doc-

trines of Rome. His own opinion regarding the cause of the complaints from the younger Puritan Fellows was that they represented "mere quarrels of envie against their rulers." It is recorded that with Dr. Caius' death shortly afterwards "all the remainder of his days were embittered."

Nearer to our own time, President James Madison of the United States was treated for a progressive condition of rheumatoid arthritis by Dr. Robley Dunglison for many years. By 1832 he reported that the shoulders, wrists, fingers, and feet of his patient were crippled, and that the President was laid upon a settee for business interviews. The patient wrote in the same year: "My fingers make smaller letters and my feet make smaller steps, but my heart survives." His periodical exacerbations were treated with strict starvation. It is reported that he had to engage a special secretary to deal with the flood of "cures" which he received daily from all parts of the world.

Still closer, and in another sphere, we remember that the great French painter, Renoir, suffered increasingly from rheumatoid arthritis from 1897 until his death in 1919. His last years were spent in such agony that his relatives considered that suicide would have offered a pardonable release; but in spite of this he continued to paint until within a few hours of his death. It is said that even critical expert assessment of his work will show remarkably little evidence of the crippled condition of his hands and wrists.

Treatment

The treatment of rheumatoid arthritis has, until the last few years, been empirical. This was inevitable in view of the almost complete ignorance of its nature and origins, whilst observation that the nervous system appeared to be involved often led to a preference for dramatic methods. The words of Sydenham, written in 1683, remain true of some forms of treatment even today. He said of the elaborate and exhausting methods to which many patients had been subjected that such antics were certainly capable of exercising a remarkable effect upon a patient; but it seemed to him doubtful that the majority would produce any effect upon the disease. In this he may have been influenced by Sir Francis Bacon who wrote in his *Essays* (1597) that: "Some physicians are so regular in proceeding according to art for this disease that they respect not sufficiently the condition of the patient."

Modern "folk-lore" prescribes a multiplicity of infallible cures amongst which may be mentioned such hardy annuals as: the juice of a lemon in hot water on waking, fresh fruit juice with epsom salts, barley water, spiritual healing, washing soda in the bath water, sulphur in the socks, honey and cider vinegar, bicarbonate of soda in milk, mud and foam baths, acupuncture, whisky and camphor massage, bicycling, and horse-back riding, to mention only a selection.

Physical Exercise

Both exercise and rest in varying degrees and forms have always been advocated. Hippocrates gave up-to-date advice for the use of chronic arthritics whose hands were affected: "In such cases of arthritis it is well to give the patients wax to knead with the fingers, and weights to hold in the hands, and afterwards to swing. Later as the patient improves, they should be made heavier." He stressed the advantage of active over passive exercises: "For lack of exercise, when the patient has been immobile a long while, the joints become weak . . . the joints are affected for the reason that the sinews and muscles have become weakened."

Sydenham strongly advocated physical exercise for the chronic arthritic, as also for the sufferer with gout. Soon several ingenious machines were introduced whereby the action of horseback riding could be simulated without leaving the house. And in 1704 Dr. Francis Fuller introduced the idea of remedial exercises much as we know them today, in a book entitled *Medicina Gymnastica,* whose sub-title was "Or a treatise concerning the power of exercise with respect to the animal economy, and the greater necessity of it in the cure of several Distempers."

Cullen said, in *First Lines of the Practice of Physic* (1776) that he felt that: "The chief cure of the chronic rheumatism is to be expected of external remedies. Of these heat is the chief, being that which sets the whole processes of the body going . . . but this may be hurtful if improperly applied." He also devoted considerable space to consideration of the use of movements and of friction; the latter he considered could most conveniently be produced with the aid of the flesh-brush. This was a type of large scrubbing brush with bristles of light whalebone, to be used either by itself or in conjunction with the infrequent ritual of a hot bath. He also advocated an occasional course of sulphur baths, such as were to be found in the nearby Scottish spa of Strathpether.

Rest

It was not until 1863 that the intelligent use of rest was discussed authoritatively. In that year John Hilton, surgeon to Guy's Hospital, published his celebrated book, *Rest and Pain.* In this he pointed out the necessity of resting joints inflamed with arthritis, this being nature's method of cure, and pain her method of securing that rest. He pointed out, however, that in common with many of nature's good ideas, "this device is but imperfectly adapted for its end . . . the response to an abnormal stimulus being never so perfectly adapted as the response to a normal one." If this were so, as he sensibly pointed out, the abnormal mechanism would, in the course of evolution, replace the normal. "So man must study to improve upon Nature's lead."

The degree in which both local and general rest is most beneficial in this disease is still a matter of learned discussion. It has been said of Hilton's methods that a generation of doctors who rested nearly everything too much produced more than a generation of crippled rheumatoid arthritics. On the other hand Dr. Robert Bridges, a physician at St. Bartholomew's Hospital who afterwards became the Poet Laureate of England, reported (1876) that he felt considerable satisfaction with the success of multiple splinting in acute and chronic arthritis, and drew the attention of his colleagues to the work of Otto Heubner of Leipzig (1871) who had popularised this method in Germany, and his predecessor in the same field, Professor Concato of Bologna. In the United States the credit of pioneering the use of light plaster splintage to relieve pain and prevent deformity in rheumatoid arthritis must go to Loring Swain of Boston (1934).

The sole early reference I have found to the nursing care of patients who are crippled with this disease is that of S. A. Tissot, the Professor of Physic in Lausanne, who said in his little book, *Advice with Regard to Health* (translation 1793): "We may save these sick a good deal of pain by putting one strong towel always under their back, and another under their thighs, in order to move them the more easily. Later, when their hands are without pain, a third towel hung upon a cord which is fastened across the bed will assist them in moving themselves."

Electricity

Such treatment is far from modern. As an early example we may consider the report of the Roman physician, Scribonius Largus. He was wont to bring his arthritic patients to the beach of Ostia, near Rome, and place their feet upon a torpedo fish, one of the formidable Mediterranean Ray family. When the tide came up a considerable shock of static electricity was delivered, which Scribonius asserted led to several permanent cures. Interest in this somewhat unusual technique was revived by John Hunter's trial and description of the electric organ of this fish, following the reports of the discoveries of Galvani and Volta, in the eighteenth century. The first modern reference to the use of electricity for arthritis is contained in a lecture delivered by William Cullen in Edinburgh in 1766, who said that "it appeared to be a very powerful stimulus to the sanguinous system, as also to the nerves . . . hence I have ordered it in many cases of chronic rheumatism." Failure he thought might result either "from not applying it for a sufficient time . . . some have required months"; or "from not using a sufficient degree of it."

On the lay side the enthusiastic Reverend John Wesley, founder of Methodism, wrote a small book, *The Desideratum, or Electricity Made Plain and Useful* (1759), in which he mentioned, amongst many other diseases suitable for this new method, several cases of gout and arthritis which were quite cured "by setting them on Rosin while one drew sparks from the diseased parts." It has been said that he established a small free dispensary for such treatment. This may have led to a static therapeutic electrical machine being installed for the use of patients in the Middlesex Hospital in 1797, at a cost of less than five guineas; and a larger one in St. Bartholomew's Hospital ten years later. After Michael Faraday had developed his induction coil "Faradic" therapy was also employed, much in the form in which we use it today, largely by Julius Althous (1833–1900) of King's College Hospital, London.

Quacks

The introduction of such mysterious forces as magnetism and electricity were naturally seized upon avidly by the quacks. The most celebrated of these was Elisha Perkins, born in 1741 in Connecticut. There he patented his "Celebrated Metallic Tractors," and made an easy fortune; George Washington is said to have purchased a pair. He then sent his son to London, where he also was so successful that a Perkinsean Institute, under the patronage of Earl Rivers and a committee of noblemen and gentlemen (which included Benjamin Franklin's son) was set up so that he could the more easily be consulted. His tractors consisted in a pair of metal compasses whose points were of different metals and about the size and shape of a pencil. The cure resulted from the "affinity they have with the offending matter which will be drawn out." This method was "effective for all arthritic, gouty and rheumatic pains, both acute and chronic, including the toothache [which at this time was regarded as arthritis of the dental socket], as well as paralysis—either in men or horses." Perkins was discredited finally by Dr. John Haygarth, who reported (1810) exactly similar results obtained in Bath Hospital with "a pair of painted

wooden tractors and a sufficiency of verbal mumbo-
jumbo."

The poet, Crabbe, himself a doctor, musing upon the
gullibility of those distinguished circles from which it
has always seemed that the quacks may obtain unlimited
patronage, wrote:

> From powerful causes spring the empirics' claims;
> Man's love of life, his weaknesses and pains.
> These first induce him the vile trash to try,
> Then lend his name—that other men may buy.

Through the next hundred years electricity still seemed
to the quacks a fertile field. Such advertisements as the
following (1862) could be found in every paper: "*Medical
Galvanism*—After being galvanised for four weeks a man
who was an invalid confined to bed for months came to
Mr. Harthill of 65 Princes Street, Edinburgh, a perfect
object with rheumatism, and left him freed from all his
pains and able to walk many miles in a day." Electric
belts and corsets were sold for high prices, and "mag-
netic" rings and amulets came into fashion again. Several
respectable fortunes in the United States are said to have
originated in this remunerative "trade."

The belief that untreated rheumatoid arthritis will
inevitably "burn itself out" dies hard, and it was no
doubt this which led Sir William Osler, who had no
great interest in this field of medicine, to say in one of
his more iconoclastic utterances that his favourite prescription for this disease was: "Time and hope in equal
and divided doses." During the "enlightened" postwar
period, 1920–1935, a host of remedies for rheumatoid arthritis were introduced amid popular acclaim. Today
they are mostly already forgotten. Of these we may recall
the removal of hypothetical foci of infection, treatment

by protein shock, vaccines controlled with the "opsonic index," bee venom, fever therapy, sulphur injections in many forms, and Professor Bier's method of passive congestion of the joints with a rubber bandage.

Medicinal remedies

Effective medicinal remedies, other than salicylates, have only been available since Forestier in France, although reasoning upon a false analogy, introduced successfully (1929) the periodical injection of salts of gold into the muscles of sufferers. Next came the momentous introduction of the steroid hormones by Philip Hench of the Mayo Clinic. The rapid, although ephemeral effect, of large doses upon patients crippled with rheumatoid arthritis was dramatically demonstrated in 1949 in New York before a large international medical audience. In the next year, with his collaborator E. C. Kendall, he received the Nobel Prize. These derivatives of cortisone, or ACTH—substances which are normally formed in the adrenal or pituitary glands—have the unique property of reversing the process of inflammation, whatever its cause, for so long as the affected tissues remain under their influence. This is not a cure; but physiological suppressives of this nature had never previously been available. Under the influence of such substances, which are now manufactured synthetically, rheumatoid arthritis can be induced to go into remission in a considerable proportion of cases.

More recently other types of synthetic anti-inflammatory drugs, unconnected with cortisone, mostly of the phenylbutazone group, have been developed and will often also give great relief; and an important addition to our understanding of the correct management of rheumatoid arthritis has resulted over the last twenty years from the work of Hans Selye of Toronto, and others, by the recognition of the relevance of emotional and stress factors in its causation.

The search for a truly curative agent for this disease continues. Such an agent will need to arrest the disease at whatever stage it has reached, and so prevent any further progress, if it is to fulfil our hopes. With accumulating knowledge we need no longer subscribe to Sydenham's opinion: "as to a radical cure, one altogether perfect, and one whereby a patient might be freed from even the disposition to disease—this lies, like Truth, at the bottom of a well. . . ."

Research

If a final cure—or better still, prevention—is to be achieved, as no doubt it will, intensive research into the origins of the disease is required. An increasing volume has been undertaken during the past twenty years in most countries. Although no single great discovery has yet emerged clues seem to be pointing in the direction of that fascinating field of scientific knowledge known as auto-immunity, whose first cultivator was Sir McFarlane Burnet, head of the great Research Institute in Melbourne, Australia. It was as early as 1930 that suspicion formed that a reaction of this nature might play a significant role in the causation of rheumatoid arthritis. In 1948 the so-called specific "rheumatoid factor" was isolated from the blood of sufferers, and the well-known Rose-Waaler diagnostic test, which employs this factor, was devised. The rheumatoid factor is currently thought to be an anti-body to the gamma globulin in the sufferer's own body, and its presence certainly indicates some important disturbance of his immune mechanisms.

The other main field in which advance seems likely is

that of genetics. We may remember that William Heberden suspected that rheumatoid arthritis was often a familial complaint, whilst Sir Charles Scudamore quoted in his book (1816) the old observation that the "sons of gouty fathers may develop the gout; but their more delicate daughters will tend to suffer with the rheumatic arthritis." These early incursions into genetics were quoted with approbation by Dr. F. J. Poynton (1900) who predicted, rightly, that this subject would shortly absorb much interest in the modern generation of medical scientists. It is the enormous recent technical advances in this discipline which largely renders work in the field of rheumatology so hopeful. As we now know the influence of genetic functions upon the body economy is legion, and the ways in which they can modify our susceptibility to the disease are incalculable.

During the last few years a new technique has developed, mostly in England, whereby from the statistical study of large groups of patients the clinical and other impressions of our predecessors can be evaluated and up-to-date theories of causation tested. These population surveys are now beginning to contribute substantially to our knowledge and understanding of rheumatoid and other rheumatic diseases.

Attempts to measure the social and economic importance of rheumatoid arthritis are of recent origin. The first survey of this type was by Kahlmeter of Sweden in 1923. This was rapidly followed by the famous report on the rheumatic diseases drafted by J. A. Glover for the British Ministry of Health in 1924 which first drew the attention of the English-speaking world to the importance of this field of medicine. It was shown that a sixth of the industrial incapacity of the country was accounted for by "rheumatism" and arthritis, and the approximate enormous cost of such disability was assessed. This proved a salutary stimulus which initiated subsequent world-wide interest in rheumatoid arthritis and other diseases of the rheumatic group. This eventually resulted in the foundation of the Empire Rheumatism Council. Modern American rheumatology can be said to have started officially on March 17, 1946, when the American Committee for the Control of Rheumatism was founded at a meeting in the Racquet Club in Philadelphia, which had been called by Dr. Ralph Pemberton, "to create an interest in a neglected field." This developed in time into the American Rheumatism Association, and by 1948 money had become available for research through the formation of the Arthritis and Rheumatism Association. Since then intense study is constantly being directed towards detecting and ravelling the complex interplay of factors—genetic, metabolic, infective, immunological, or constitutional in origin—which constitute this disease.

Thus, although the cause of rheumatoid arthritis has not yet been discovered, the contributions from these and other research fields are serving to confirm on a sure basis the historical belief of Garrod and other earlier observers, that rheumatoid arthritis is a separate disease entity with entirely independent status in the rheumatic field—and can be conquered.

CHAPTER X

Ankylosing Spondylitis

This disease, although not very common, is important as it affects chiefly apparently healthy young men and, if it remains unchecked, it results in complete "poker back" stiffness and often considerable crippling of the limbs and chest. In view of its striking nature it is curious that so few specific records of this disease were found in medical literature until a few years ago. During the last world war the Air Force medical authorities instituted a routine investigation of all recruits who complained of backache or "lumbago." The results showed that sacro-iliitis, the premonitory stage of ankylosing spondylitis, is a more commonly occurring phenomenon than had previously been believed. It seems probable, however, that a proportion of such cases are self-limiting and do not progress beyond that stage.

Evidence of its existence thousands of years before Christ exists in the Egyptian and Nubian skeletons unearthed by Sir Grafton Elliot Smith during his tenure of the Chair of Anatomy in Cairo (1908), of which a pictorial record exists in the British Museum; and also later by his colleague Sir Marc Ruffer (1918), the Professor of Bacteriology.

Hippocrates mentioned an arthritis in which "the vertebrae of the spine and neck may be affected with the pain, and it extends to the os sacrum." He described the occurrence of joint ankylosis, and said that "the humour is difficult to dissolve and is thick, white and like an hailstone." This may refer to spondylitis.

In Lucian's play, the *Ocypus*, written in the second century, the finale may be thought relevant to our theme: the athletic young hero arrogantly mocked his arthritic seniors. The goddess, Podagra, indignant at this, set one of her torments onto his feet. Such was his courage, however, that he was able to pretend that he felt no pain. So the angry goddess sent others onto his back. This was successful, and he was laid low forever.

In the fifth-century work by the Byzantine physician, Caelius Aurelianus, called *De Ischiadicis et Psoadicis*, mention was made of a number of conditions which partially correspond to the clinical picture of this disease. He referred, for instance, to a stiff woodenness of the attachments of the lower part of the vertebral column: "The patient is afflicted with pain in the nates, moves slowly, and can only bend or stand erect with difficulty" (Mettler 1947).

After this the next specific mention of spondylitis would seem to be in Book XV of the posthumous *De Re Anatomica* (1559) by the celebrated sixteenth-century anatomist, Realdo Colombo, successor to Vesalius at Padua and a friend of Michelangelo, which was recently brought to my notice by Professor O'Malley of the University of California. In this Colombo described the interesting variations from the normal which he had encountered during a lifetime of dissecting. He was one of the first anatomists whose knowledge of the normal structure of the body would have been sufficient to do this with confidence. Speaking of spondylitis he said:

> In the Papal Palace there is now to be seen a lower jaw from the head of a giant—for it is the largest head I ever saw—in which this jaw is so firmly fused to the head that all movement is lacking, and was so during life. Furthermore I saw with my own eyes that a vertebra was so attached

to the occiput that it also could not move at all . . . Also
I saw the femur united with the tibia and the patella.

He then described the union of the os ilium to the
sacrum, which is now known to be the usual initial lesion
in this disease.

Later he described an even more convincing case:

> That excellent physician Giovanni Bertoni of Lariccia, a
> very good friend of mine, gave me a skeleton which I care-
> fully preserved at home for the instruction of my students.
> In this all the bones, that is to say all the joints of the body
> from head to extremities as far as the toes of the feet, are
> seen to be united; four teeth are lacking in it, two above
> and two below, in that region where food and drink had to
> be introduced. The patient had lived for a long time in
> Rome in the Hospital of the Incurables. . . . He could
> move nothing except his eyes, tongue, penis, and abdomen.
> Also the thorax—for the cartilages articulated to the ribs
> had not yet coalesced; the remaining parts of his body and
> spine completely lacked motion.

In the works of the great English physician, Thomas
Sydenham, we find a description of what he called "rheumatic lumbago," of which he stated:

> It is properly called the rheumatical ache of the loins, a
> violent pain being fixed there, and stretching often to the
> Os Sacrum . . . upon which account I have heretofore been
> mistaken, thinking it was produced by gravel sticking in
> those parts; whereas in truth it owed its use to the peccant
> and inflammed matter of that *Rheumatism* which afflicts
> only those parts, the rest of the body being untouched. The
> severe pain continues as the other species (chronic rheuma-
> tism) if it be not cured after the same manner; grievously
> afflicting the poor Patient so that he cannot lie in his Bed,
> but is forced to leave it or to sit upright at nights, rocking
> himself continually.

As O'Connell pointed out (1956), Sydenham invariably
confined himself to clinical descriptions. It was not until

the next century that Morgagni developed the system of correlating clinical with post-mortem findings in disease, and so initiating scientific medicine.

It was, however, the short-lived Irish genius, Bernard Connor (1666?–1698), who generally receives priority for the first pathological account of ankylosing spondylitis, in his M.D. thesis (Rheims 1691), which he entitled briefly *Une Dissertation Physique sur la Continuité de Plusieurs Os, a l'Occasion d'une Fabrique Surprenante d'un Tronc de Squelette Humain, ou les Vertèbres, les Côtes, l'Os Sacrum, et les Os des Iles, qui Naturellement sont Distincts et Séparez, ne font qu'un Seul Os Continu et Inséparable.* In this he described in detail a skeleton showing the advanced stage of this disease and reconstructed with some accuracy the patient's probable symptoms during life. He also made a few wild surmises as to its causes. This thesis he later expanded and published in the *Philosophical Transactions of the Royal Society* (1695).

Connor lived in Ireland until he was twenty years old, when the "wanderlust" led him abroad to study medicine, and to the situation of tutor to the two sons of the High Chancellor of Poland whom he met in France and with whom he travelled through Europe. On their return to Poland he was appointed physician to the monarch, King Jan Sobietski, until he returned to London in 1695 where he rapidly became a Fellow of both the Royal Society and the Royal College of Physicians. He died in the parish of St. Giles-in-the-Fields, probably of malaria, a convert to the Church of England, with his servant and the Rector of the parish barring the door to the two Roman priests who had been sent to "rectify" this untimely change of faith.

Percival Pott, F.R.S., of St. Bartholomew's Hospital,

John Hunter's teacher in surgery, published in 1779 a work called *Remarks on that Kind of Palsy of the Lower Limbs which is Frequently Found to Accompany a Curvature of the Spine.* This was the first description of tuberculous spondylitis, or Pott's disease, a condition which can be confused with the ankylosing type.

In 1741 Robert, Bishop of Cork, in a letter written to the Earl of Egmont, had given an excellent description of a skeleton in the museum of Trinity College, Dublin, in which the spine and most other joints showed complete ankylosis, evidently an example of true ankylosing spondylitis. Stiffness of the back had occurred at the age of 18, and ankylosis of all his limbs gradually occurred: "The only use he was capable of being put to was that of watchman, as once he was fixed in his station it was impossible for him to desert it. He is one entire bone from the top of his head to his ankles. . . ." This preparation was referred to by Philip M. Lyons in an article in the *Lancet* (1831), in which he also described the case of a Dubliner, aged thirty-six, who had suffered with this disease for seven and a half years. With the hope of obtaining a post-mortem examination Lyons admitted the man into his hospital, and unwisely gave a clinical demonstration shortly afterwards. The man's suspicions were aroused by the interest which was shown at this, so he decided to discharge himself home, where he died. His friends, in accordance with his written instructions, then cut up his body into small pieces in order to outwit the pathologist. However, a year later Lyons had managed to obtain these and, from them, reconstructed the complete skeleton!

Throughout the nineteenth century a number of distinguished medical men published isolated observations and examples of this disease. These notably included

R. B. Todd, F.R.S., and Sir Benjamin Brodie, the King's Sergeant-Surgeon, to whom Robert Adams dedicated his *Treatise on the Rheumatic Gout* (1857): "In testimony of the benefit he has rendered . . . by his successful efforts to improve our knowledge . . . of diseases of the joints." In this Adams described the syndrome of ankylosing spondylitis, recognised the typical sex incidence, but considered the condition to be merely a variant of rheumatoid arthritis, as do some authorities still, particularly in the United States. Brodie had written a small book entitled *Observations on Diseases of the Joints* (1818) based upon his practical experience at St. George's Hospital. This work may be said to have introduced the study of bone pathology to the academic world. Without knowledge of the aetiology of the various conditions he describes, he was nonetheless able to distinguish between caries (tuberculosis) and "caries of other sorts. . . . In the latter," he said, "suppuration does not occur, and the pathology starts not in the bone but around the intervertebral cartilages, thus giving rise to a gradual curve of the spine and not angulation."

In this volume Sir Benjamin described the case history of a boy suffering with ankylosing spondylitis and its common accompaniment, iritis; perhaps the first published record of this association. He noted the tendency to exacerbations and remissions, and later commented on the post-mortem appearances in that "the bodies of a greater or smaller number of vertebrae are firmly ankylosed, there being at the same time a deposit of bony matter here and there on the surface adhering to the bone beneath, and extending from one vertebra to the other. It is reasonable to suppose," he continues, "that such a change in the condition of the spine must have been the result of a long-continued inflammation."

Reiter's Disease

He also described for the first time a case of arthritis
of the spine whose onset was associated with a genital
discharge and severe conjunctivitis, an association which
is nowadays erroneously designated Reiter's disease. We
know that the urethritis in these cases is of a non-venereal
type, but it is interesting to note that he also was aware
that it was not the result of gonorrhoeal infection, as his
description starts as follows: "A gentleman forty-five years
of age, in the middle of June 1817 became affected with
symptoms *resembling* those of gonorrhoea. There was a
purulent discharge. . . ." His patient soon developed
pain in the joints of his feet, and later conjunctivitis.
Six months later he suffered a recurrence of the syndrome
which lasted six weeks. His treatment included blisters to
the knees, leeches, and *Vinum colchici,* which Brodie considered very helpful. Six years later Sir Astley Cooper of
St. Thomas' Hospital described a similar case in the
Lancet. Reiter's disease—this triad of arthritis, urethritis,
and conjunctivitis—derives its name from the description
of such a case published nearly one hundred years later
(1916) by Hans Reiter, a Lieutenant serving in the German Army Medical Corps on the Balkan front. He
wrongly believed the causative agent to be a spirochaete
which he had isolated from the patient's stool.

Samuel Hare, the orthopaedic surgeon at Leeds (1849),
Holmes Coste (1867), "a cautious and discriminating
surgeon" who, we are told, however, died at his house in
London "entertaining delusions of unbounded wealth,"
and H. P. C. Wilson of Philadelphia (1856) described
cases of ankylosing spondylitis. The last-named's patient
was a negress—a most unusual circumstance—whilst
Bernard E. Broadhurst (1858) described the progress of

two cases of typical spondylitis which followed gonococcal infection and which he referred to as "rheumatism
of the spine." It was C. Hilton Fagge, nephew of John
Hilton of Guy's Hospital, and surgeon to the same hospital, who contributed in 1877 his classical account of
the disease and post-mortem findings to the *Transactions of the Pathological Society of London*. This has
generally received favourable comparison with those of
Bechterev, Strümpell, and Pierre Marie, although these
latter are more widely known.

The account given by the Russian, Vladimir Bechterev
(1893), was of five cases, and does not seem to entitle him
to the priority which the frequent attachment of his
name to this disease suggests. Indeed, it seems probable
after reading his account, that only two of these patients
can have been suffering with true spondylitis.

Strümpell gave a careful description (1897) of three
cases examined by him in Leipzig, and his name is still
generally attached to the disease in his country. But it
would appear to be the Frenchman, Pierre Marie, Professor of Neurology in the University of Paris in succession
to Jean Charcot, who best merits eponymous fame in this
connection.

Marie was born in 1853, his mother being only sixteen
at the time, and died in 1940. Whilst assistant to Charcot
in 1886, they examined together a patient whose spine
was completely rigid and were unable to make a diagnosis. Marie always made full methodical notes on his
cases, so when he came across a similar patient ten years
later, and shortly afterwards a further one, he studied
them intensively and in 1898 published his paper, *La
Spondylose Rhizomélique,* in which he described practically every feature of ankylosing spondylitis which today
we recognise as being of importance. These included the

typical gait, the flattened lumbar spine, and the bowing forward of the neck and chest which, with the flexion of the hips and knees, create in profile the outline of a Z. Without the advantages of X-ray or post-mortem examination he described the complete fusion of the spine, chest, and hips, and mentioned the consequent difficulty in breathing and walking. He recognised the predilection of the disease for teen-age males, and denied that venereal infection played a part in its origin. His work was well carried on by his pupil and successor, André Léri, who completed the pathological descriptions from post-mortem material from these cases.

Pierre Marie was also the first to describe acromegaly, as well as that curious condition sometimes encountered by rheumatologists known as hypertrophic pulmonary osteoarthropathy. This consists in an enlargement and "clubbing" of the terminal finger joints which is generally associated with chronic disease of the chest.

J. E. Goldthwait of Boston wrote a comprehensive article (1899) distinguishing what was evidently ankylosing spondylitis from the various senile spinal changes with which it was, and is, sometimes confused. Unfortunately, however, he referred to it throughout as osteoarthritis of the spine, and therefore minimised the influence of his opinions.

Thus, to summarise the highlights of the story of ankylosing spondylitis, Caelius Aurelianus and Sydenham would seem to share the honours of being the earliest authors to have mentioned this disease; Bernard Connor (1695) was the first to give an account of the late skeletal changes, but unfortunately he never, so far as we know, saw a live sufferer. Benjamin Brodie (1850) appears to have been the first fully to have correlated the pathologi-

cal appearances with the clinical picture, although Lyons
had described a case in clinical detail which he ener-
getically followed beyond the grave. The subject was
only written large onto the map of clinical medicine,
however, during the nineteenth century with the advent
of Fagge, Bechterev, Strümpell, and Marie; and the
greatest of these was Marie.

Treatment

If we search the literature for the methods of treatment which were employed in such cases we get little
help until this century, except for several descriptions of
formidable "spinal supports" which it is hard to believe
could have been worn even by the most docile patient.
John Hilton refers to this disease in his *Rest and Pain*
(1863). He says that complete rest "will generally result
in a complete cure . . . but ankylosis will generally be
found to be complete!"

Sir Richard Quain, in his *Dictionary of Medicine*
(1882), a standard work, had nothing further to contribute, except that: "If anchylosis has taken place in an
incomplete degree an attempt may be made to restore
mobility by forceful or gradual extension, by passive
motion, or by massage."

Spa treatment (hydrotherapy) became deservedly popular towards the beginning of the present century, and in
the late nineteen-twenties deep X-ray treatment was introduced by Gilbert Scott and others. Such treatment was
found to be effective in suppressing the activity of the
disease and in relieving its pain, but has fallen under a
cloud of recent years owing to the suspicion that it may
also produce harmful side effects, including possibly that
dread disease, leukaemia. Modern treatment avoids im-

mobilisation and depends largely upon the use of the new anti-inflammatory drugs such as phenylbutazone or the steroid hormones. It is very rare now to see cases of ankylosing spondylitis which have progressed to severe deformity, such as were common only thirty years ago.

CHAPTER XI

Osteoarthritis

Until a disease has been adequately identified, intelligent study of its causes or cure remains scientifically unrewarding. For this reason the field of chronic arthritis until recently tended to appeal chiefly to speculative medical scholastics and the more numerous body of quacks.

Sir Alfred Garrod was the first to differentiate chronic arthritis finally from variants of gout when he described the rheumatoid type as a separate entity in 1859. Osteoarthritis thus became recognisable by a process of exclusion and was awarded its name by John Kent Spender, a physician of Bath, in 1888, although he applied it wrongly to include other types.

Undoubtedly, however, the disease had been afflicting both man and beast from the earliest times, as we may judge from their remains. *Pithecanthropus erectus,* the famous "Java man," one of our earliest known ancestors, dating from some 500,000 years ago, is reported to have possessed an osteoarthritic hip, whilst Virchow's descriptions of neolithic remains contain many references to this condition, for which he coined the term "cave-gout." The skeletons of the ancient Roman garrison disinterred in 1962 in Yorkshire, England, were also reported to show a high proportion of osteoarthritic sufferers.

In the aphorism of Hippocrates referring to "an arthritis which seizes the great joints, which are able to contain it, but which does not usually go beyond these," it seems possible to discern the picture of osteoarthritis.

In other places he is more obviously describing cases of
tuberculous arthritis, a condition which is believed to
have been common in ancient Greece, and which was
thought to be an acute form of osteoarthritis until quite
recent times.

Tuberculous Arthritis

The earliest attempt at differentiation between this
condition and osteoarthritis is perhaps that of the fifth-
century physician Caelius Aurelianus, who divided
chronic arthritis into the hot and cold varieties. The
latter may represent tuberculous infection as he stated
that it was not subject to remissions, affected the patient's
health, lead to great wasting, and would eventually cause
his death.

The first sophisticated description of tuberculous arthritis was that of the Royalist Sergeant-Surgeon Richard
Wiseman (1622?–1676) of Exeter, who named it "the
white swelling of the joints," and correctly recognised its
"scrofulous" (tuberculous) association from the fact that
lung disease often coexisted, and the lymphatic glands of
the victims generally enlarged. He classified it as one of
the varieties of the "King's Evil," and so, he thought,
might sometimes be expected to respond favourably to
the "Ceremony of the royal touch." The condition became well recognised throughout western England and
was referred to as "the Cruells." Dr. Samuel Johnson
stated that he had been much indebted to the works of
Wiseman whilst compiling his great dictionary. He referred to them as "that mine of good surgical nomenclature." Johnson himself had been "touched" for a scrofulous condition of the neck by Queen Anne in 1712.
Pringle wrote (1752): "I remember two cases in hospital
in which hip pain was exquisite and constant and nothing

gave relief; so that the men, growing hectic, and after long pining, died in agony. From other cases I have seen since I imagine that these men had a suppuration about the hip joint."

Tuberculous arthritis had to await the birth of bacteriology, however, for full confirmation of Wiseman's accurate clinical observations. Robert Koch described his discovery of the causative bacillus of tuberculosis in 1882, and Strangeways was the first actually to culture this bacillus from an infected joint as late as 1920.

Syphilis was correctly incriminated by Jean Charcot (1825–1893) as the primary cause of that form of degenerative arthritis, indistinguishable from osteoarthritis pathologically, which results from localised atrophy occurring in the nervous system, and is now generally known as "Charcot's joint." This he announced at the London meeting of the International Congress of Medicine in 1881. The model he made in wax of his first case is still in the Salpêtrière museum. This condition although pathologically indistinguishable from degenerative osteoarthritis, progresses to far greater deformity owing to the curious lack of pain experienced by its victims in the affected joints. It may have been a joint of this nature that Realdo Colombo reported (1559) that he had seen in the course of his dissection of a knee joint: "the femur and tibia extended into an incredible swelling." Syphilis was at the height of its epidemic virulence at that time, and no doubt its manifestations were often of a florid type.

Classification and Pathology

The confusion which still in some degree surrounds the classification of arthritis may have been largely initiated by the first published attempt at systematic classi-

fication in Sauvages' *Nosologica Methodica* (1763), where
he divided gout into fourteen varieties and "rheumatisms" into ten. Osteoarthritis seems to correspond with
the division he named *rhumatismus arthriticus:* "which
affects the large joints and never exhibits gouty concretions." William Cullen, never to be outdone, improved
upon this in his classification by increasing the varieties
of rheumatism to thirty-four! It is interesting to note
that he included in a minor category toothache, of which
he says: "With some degree of propriety physicians have
ever considered the toothache as a species of rheumatism
('Dentagra'), for it affects the membranes and the sockets
of the jaws." The tooth and its socket were considered as
a primitive joint, and the toothache therefore as an arthritis.

William Heberden gave a good account of osteoarthritis in his *Commentaries* (1802) under the generic heading
of chronic rheumatism, although not unnaturally at
times he confused it with other forms of disease. This
work epitomised his accumulated medical wisdom and
was published posthumously by his son. In it we find his
celebrated remarks upon the osteoarthritic nodes of the
terminal finger joints which bear his name:

> *Digitorum Nodi:* What are these little hard knobs about
> the size of a small pea, which are frequently seen upon the
> fingers, particularly a little below the top, near the joint?
> They have no connection with the gout, being found in per-
> sons who never had it. They continue for life; and being
> hardly ever attended by pain or disposed to become sores,
> are rather unsightly than inconvenient, though they must
> be of some little hindrance to the use of the fingers.

The first person who convincingly separated the osteoarthritic from the rheumatoid type of arthritis was
Robert Adams who in his *Treatise on the Rheumatic*

Gout (1857), the first special work to be written on arthritis, stated that the two varieties could be distinguished by the predilection of the one for the small joints of the extremities, and of the other for the larger joints, "either singly or in conjunction." For osteoarthritis of the hip he coined the term "malum coxae senilis," but pointed out that its ravages were not confined to old age: "Indeed, I have observed it in sufferers under the age of twenty years." Commenting upon Heberden's nodes he described the method of formation by "small synovial cysts which become developed in the cellular tissue surrounding affected joints; the fluid is later absorbed and converted into small solid tumours." He described well the post-mortem appearance of joint cavities, and rightly believed ankylosis to be rare except in cases where infection was the cause. Within the limits of the techniques available to him, and by accurate observation and a good knowledge of the normal appearances, he can be said to have taken the subject as far as was possible at that time. The elder Garrod was able to acquit both forms from any association with gout by devising his famous thread test in 1859.

In 1904 Joel Ernest Goldthwait of Boston proposed classification of chronic arthritis based upon the appearance of the soft tissues. He spoke of the "hypertrophic" type which would correspond to osteoarthritis, the "atrophic" which was the rheumatoid type, and "infectious arthritis" which included all other clinical entities. This was "improved upon" by E. H. Nichols and F. L. Richardson (1909), who classified all chronic arthritics into the proliferative or degenerative: "Two types of a single disease." The modern distinction has evolved as the result of work by the committees appointed for this purpose by the Royal College of Physicians of London and the International League against Rheumatism.

Probably the first post-mortem report on a case of osteoarthritis was that recently found amongst the manuscripts (no. 54) of John Hunter, *An Account of the Dissection of Morbid Bodies*. This described the joints of the lower limbs of an old woman who had died in St. George's Hospital, of whose medical history he knew nothing. He found cartilaginous loose bodies in both knee joints, and one in the left ankle "of the bigness of a pea, which was attached to the ligament of the joint by a strong cord. . . . On turning down the patella I saw that the cartilage was almost eroded off; both it and the end of the femur were scored in parallel grooves." Hunter's very first communication to the *Philosophical Transactions of the Royal Society* in 1743 was entitled "On the structure and diseases of the articulating cartilages," in which he also gave the first description of the normal vascular supply to the joints. He tells us that of the first sixty-five patients who were admitted to his new hospital (St. George's) five were suffering with "severe rheumatism" which involved the hip joint.

Dr. William Falconer, who had studied at Edinburgh and Leyden before settling in Bath, commenting upon the admission figures to his hospital between the years 1785 and 1793, pointed out that "as true gout is largely confined to the upper ranks of Society," his wards contained during this period "609 patients of whom 278 were victims of hip-arthritis," often with muscle wasting. It seems probable that many of these were victims of osteoarthritis.

Both Jean Charcot (1862) and the great German pathologist Rudolf Virchow (1863) studied post-mortem appearances of patients with chronic arthritis. As was said earlier, it is unfortunate that in both cases their material was obtained from the geriatric section of their hospitals so that they were dealing only with the late results and not with active disease. This led them to conclude that both forms of non-infective chronic arthritis were merely clinical variants of the same underlying pathology, and did not constitute distinct diseases. This resulted in the adoption of the unfortunate unitarian term "arthritis deformans" as a covering label for all forms, which delayed the progress of rheumatology by fifty years.

The modern distinction between rheumatoid arthritis and osteoarthritis was only made finally by A. E. Garrod in his article in the 1907 edition of Allbutt and Rolleston's *System of Medicine*, which he based upon G. A. Bannatyne's work (1896), in which he was able to assign to both rheumatoid arthritis and osteoarthritis their proper symptomatology and pathology for the first time. It is only in the last twenty years that osteoarthritis has been discovered to be the result of a metabolic defect in the cartilage which renders it less able to withstand the effects of normal aging and extra-mechanical stresses. This abnormal constitution seems to run in certain families.

Treatment

Until quite recently treatment was no different from that considered suitable for arthritis due to chronic gout. The great Frenchman, Jean Cruveilhier (1791–1874), said of the very violent treatment often employed in his time, that its inutility seemed to him to be the least of the evils which attended it; whilst even Adams (1857) wrote that "little which can be considered satisfactory has been advanced on the important subject of its medical treatment"; and R. B. Todd (1843), that great apostle of common sense, believed that "it will never be found to be curable owing to the organic changes which take place in the bone itself." He advocated attempts to bring some relief to sufferers, however, and listed as possibilities warm baths, leeches applied locally, small doses of potassium iodide, cod-liver oil both internally and externally applied, and "Chelsea Pensioner Electuary." Rest in the early stages he thought important, and in the later phases exercises were to be encouraged. He was sceptical regarding the efficacy of spa treatment. The use of leeches locally was universal, although Pringle had warned that benefit would only be obtained from them in such pains of joints as were attended with both inflammation and fluid swelling.

Sir Thomas Watson, the author of the most renowned textbook of his time, stated (1848) that pain may often be alleviated by means of warmth and light friction around the joints. He recommended flannel underwear and hot-brine or vapour baths. Guaiacum, he thought, should constitute routine medication, with the addition of Dover's powder for pain. For those who could afford to do so he advocated removal to a warm, dry climate during cold weather.

Until the era of modern analgesics the prescription of drugs was generally thought to be less helpful in chronic osteoarthritis than in other "rheumatisms." Sir John Pringle voiced general medical opinion when he wrote (1752): "Internal medicines avail little. The best which I have tried is camphor, but not so as to force a sweat." A famous exception, however, was the "Chelsea Pensioner Electuary," devised in the eighteenth century, and still sometimes used today. It is said that Admiral Lord Anson derived so much relief from its use that he rewarded his medical practitioner with £500 and an annuity, and decreed that "this most stimulating, diaphoretick and diuretic mixture shall become available for all time" to the veterans of his and later campaigns, who had the fortune to be living in arthritic retirement in Wren's beautiful, if draughty, Royal Hospital for Old Soldiers and Sailors in the parish of Chelsea. This electuary is a somewhat nauseous treacle compounded of guaiacum, rhubarb, and sulphur.

Another more curious remedy which appeared in all the European pharmacopoeias of the seventeenth and eighteenth centuries was the impressive-sounding "Oleum Philosophorum," called in the English editions by the more prosaic and accurate appellation "Oil of Bricks." This was made by heating building bricks to red heat, and quenching them rapidly to saturation point with olive oil. They were then ground up and the powder heated in a retort "until a distillate of oil and spirit is obtained." This final product could be used either internally or externally for the cure of chronic arthritis and other complaints.

About 1850 E. C. Lasègue of Paris introduced tincture of iodine for the treatment of osteoarthritis, both by mouth and externally. Orally he recommended one drop to be taken in wine three times daily, increasing this by the same amount each day to a maximum of fifteen drops, and then down the scale again in the same way. This often appeared to help, and *faut de mieux* remained popular.

With the introduction of aspirin in 1899 a new era in comfort opened for the osteoarthritic, whilst more recently the synthesis of the phenylbutazone group of compounds renders life still more bearable for large numbers of sufferers with this painful complaint.

Spa Treatment

It had been known from early times that a stiff joint could be moved more easily under water than on dry land. Warm bathing had therefore been prescribed for arthritic patients in Greece, Rome, and Egypt. In Rome certain slaves were trained to give massage subsequently.

At Salerno where the first medical school was established in Europe, physicians continued in the twelfth century to recommend spa treatment for such patients. The places selected were those where natural mineral and sulphur or brine waters abounded such as Acqui and Abano in Italy, and Aix and La Bourboulle in France, which are still used for a similar purpose. It was the hot sulphur water which was used, however, and not the mud as today. The first authoritative publication on this subject was a collection of treatises entitled *De Balneis*, which appeared in Venice in 1553. Although the authors agreed that most patients would benefit, it was thought wise to relate a cautionary tale of how that Most Puissant Prince, the Noble Marquis d'Este, was sent to Acqui for treatment of his gout. Unfortunately he returned "with his pains ten times more agonising," and his physician was adequately disciplined for having promised more than he could perform. At this time the waters were generally taken internally as well as being administered externally.

During the eighteenth century spa treatment became highly organised in England, notably at Bath, and osteoarthritic cripples, as well as those seeking general improvement in their health, flocked there. Dr. William Cullen commented (1769) favourably upon the results of such treatment, but ever practical, added that those who cannot afford to go to such places need not despair as "I have known cases where the assiduous use of the common hot bath for a similar space of time has been equally serviceable in the chronic arthritis."

During the next century spas opened all over Europe, and the rich and the rheumatic flocked to them annually. At places such as Aix, Baden-Baden, Vichy, Wiesbaden, and Homberg, hydrotherapy was brought to a high level, whilst other ingenious methods of additional physical therapy were added to the original regime of bathing and "taking the waters." It was in pursuance of this latter objective that physiotherapy and medical electrical therapy became developed towards the end of the century, both in the spas and in town centres.

Operative Treatment

Until sixty years ago orthopaedic surgery was little more than a name and an aspiration. Pioneers such as Sir Robert Jones of Liverpool, J. E. Goldthwait of Boston, and later Reginald Watson-Jones of London, started to apply its principles to the surgical treatment of osteoarthritic joints. These principles, in chronological order of enunciation, were the correction of deformity, redistribution of body weight with the help of apparatus and shoes, arthrodesis, and arthroplasty. The last term implies the creation of an artificial joint to replace the defective natural one. The Frenchman, Jean Judet, first proposed the substitution of the head of the femur by a plastic reproduction, whilst M. N. Smith-Petersen of Boston started to experiment in 1925 with his widely used cup-arthroplasty, whereby the socket of the hip joint is replaced by a metallic cup within which the head of the femur can articulate. Such procedures are now standard usage in certain circumstances, but research into still better methods continues.

Conclusion

In discussion of a disease about which even now we
know comparatively little, and in which we are still sometimes able to give so little effective help, it may prove
rewarding to inquire into the empirical experiences of an
intelligent patient. The late E. F. Benson, son of an Archbishop of Canterbury, was a celebrated and witty scholar
who published an amusing autobiography entitled *Final
Edition* (1940). In this he chronicled the progress of his
osteoarthritic hip and its reactions to contemporary treatments, both orthodox and otherwise. His account seems
so unfortunately typical of the experience of his generation in this field that permission has graciously been given
for an extract to be quoted here.

"Most people of middle age," he says, "are liable to
rheumatic twinges, and though disquisitions on ailments
are apt to be boring, I take that risk in the hope that my
long experience (I celebrate the completion of twenty
glorious years of crippling processes very soon) may divert
or encourage other wayfarers on that dreary road." He
continues:

> These twinges much annoyed me, for I had been a skilled
> and active denizen of skating rinks and golf links and tennis
> courts, impervious to fatigue, and I regarded such threat-
> ened limitations as an offence against the liberty of the
> subject. So I hastened to consult an eminent general practi-
> tioner who after flexings and extensions solemnly bound a
> strip of adhesive plaster round the troublesome hip joint,
> which came off in my bath. I knew he used suggestion with
> his patients, and concluded that this was an appeal to my
> mind. But my mind must have been in an unreceptive
> mood: the treatment had no effect.
>
> It would be as tedious to follow the progress of this re-
> pulsive ailment as it was to suffer it. Like a clock of which

the long pointer remains stationary till a minute is completed, it paused and then registered a perceptible advance.
Activity diminished, and pain, which I abominate, increased. Firmly resolved to get rid of it, I scoured the medical cantonments of London. I went alike to notable regular
physicians and to quacks. I returned to my friend of the
sticking-plaster, who now advised tonics and a liberal consumption of oranges. He said there was no need to take an
X-ray because he knew what it would show. Another gave
me a course of atophan; another colonized my colon with
hordes of the Bacillus Bulgaricus. When that region (such
was the strategy) was securely held by this admirable Army
Corps, they would march and manoeuvre and inflict crush-
ing defeats on the injurious bacilli of disease. I took great
interest in this war. For two years I was a very diligent
Colonial Minister, and kept adding brigades of Bacillus
Bulgaricus to my garrisons, but they never seemed to win
a single engagement. Another doctor injected something
radio-active into my thigh; another some potion of dead
bacilli into my arm. Another drove iodine into the hip by
means of an electric current; another prescribed a course of
iodine taken internally in increasing doses up to the maximum, and then in diminished doses, till I arrived at the
precise point, in every sense, at which I had started. Another prescribed massage, another a system of physical exercises. I wallowed in brown mud, I drank the waters of Bath,
I floated on the buoyant and saline streams of Droitwich,
and had some healthy teeth extracted. I had a course of
intensive X-ray, alone in a room full of shining black pipes
and buzzing mechanisms; it was like figuring in some night-
mare picture by Syme. Never in my life have I pursued a
quest with such unfaltering devotion. The zeal of the Lords
of Harley Street ate me up.

The quacks, if I may call them so without libel, were
equally enterprising and empirical. I took herbal teas and
sat in tepid baths. For a long time I wore a band of small
crystals, which I take to have been glass, round my neck,
and "radio-active pads," which I take to have been flannel,
over my hips, for both were now giving trouble. I carried

a little tubular cardboard case, hermetically sealed and very heavy for its size, in my trouser pocket. One day I dropped it on the floor, the case was fractured and inside a small bottle of quicksilver. I had a course—perhaps I ought to class this among scientific treatments—of Christian Science. The healer, a most charming fellow, gave me something by Mrs. Eddy to read, while he tuned in as it were, by dipping into her textbook *Christian Science and the Key to the Scriptures*. He then closed his book and gave me mental treatment, that is to say, he absorbed himself in the conviction that disease had not any real existence, with special application to me. I warned him that I was not yet a convert, but he said that did not matter; faithless folk, who had a false claim that they were ill, could be cured just as well as believers. This astonished me for I had understood that in the miracles of healing recorded in the Gospels the faith of the patient was a condition of his cure.

These treatments overlapped; I might be wearing my radio-active pads at Droitwich or my necklace at Bath. They all ran the same course, cradled in high optimism and gently expiring in complete failure. Doubtless this abridged catalogue of them gives the impression that I was a most credulous patient to spend so much time and money on regimes which my reasonable mind rejected as rubbish. But I wanted to get well, and was prepared to do anything, however preposterous, in search of this consummation. Indeed I think it would have been very foolish not to have been so foolish, for who could tell? From time to time these practitioners cheered me up by telling me that I was walking more easily, which was not the case, for when at last one of them suggested that an X-ray skiagraph should be taken, it showed osteoarthritis in an advanced stage, and irreparable damage already done.

If this extract from Mr. Benson's autobiography seems to give a gloomy, albeit reasonably accurate, account of the plight of an osteoarthritic sufferer during the first quarter of the present century, what of the future? Research progresses in centres of learning, both in Great

Britain and the United States, and hypotheses based upon experimental work regarding this disease are being actively explored. For instance, it has been demonstrated that in mice osteoarthritis is a genetically governed disorder in which many genes are involved, whilst in women that localised form of the disease known as Heberden's nodes has now also been put on to a similar basis since its inheritance has been shown to depend upon a Mendelian dominant factor.

All this means that medical scientists at last regard this disease as an important subject for serious study; we have moved beyond the "Act of God" era, and progress in treatment, and perhaps even prevention, will follow. Surgical methods of dealing with joints damaged beyond the power of medicine to heal are also becoming more efficient and more widely disseminated. For the first time in history the future looks reasonably bright for the osteoarthritic sufferer.

CHAPTER XII

Non-Articular Rheumatism ("Fibrositis")

As has been mentioned, the ancient Greeks regarded all arthritic diseases as being the result of congestion of the affected joints, caused by an abnormal flow of one of the constituent humours of the bloodstream. The fact that this could happen to joints suggested, moreover, that it might occur in the soft tissues, the muscles, ligaments, subcutaneous tissues, and perhaps also the viscera.

Hippocrates referred to "those lighter pains which have no evident association with podagra and do not cause swellings," mentioning their unprecise localisation and character, and the fact that they tend to be weather-sensitive. He said that the stiffness, tenderness, and fatigue which they caused might be likened to that which resulted from violent exercise in the untrained athlete. This description we find elaborated by a somewhat later medical writer named Theophrastus, pupil of Aristotle and author of a celebrated book on botany. He discussed the possible site of origin of these diffuse pains, reviewing the blood vessels, the nerves, and finally the fibrous membranes and ligaments, which he considered to be the most probable source. He thought that the pains were likely to be caused by some morbid process and not as the sole result of any stress, as he noticed that this condition would often afflict very sedentary patients. He mentioned that in such people, particularly if they were obese, even light surface pressure without movement might cause considerable pain. No doubt he was describing that form

of non-articular rheumatism which we now call pannicu-
litis.

He believed all such syndromes to be due to the influx
of catarrhal humour to the fibrous tissues of the body,
causing local distention at these sites. He saw some confirmation of his theory in the fact that such pains often
accompanied general febrile catarrhal states in which an
available excess of free humour could be assumed. He
believed that localisation occurred most readily in regions which are mobile and so most liable to physical
stress and strain, such as the muscles, tendons, and synovial tissues of the weight-bearing limbs. Although he recognised that gout played no part in their genesis he postulated that sufferers must be possessed of a rheumatic
"diathesis," and that the pains could then be provoked by
general or local fatigue, either of a mental or physical
character. Accordingly he labelled this group of non-articular pains with the generic term of "lassitude." He said:
"This sensation of lassitude is a feeling of heaviness in
the organs of locomotion, such as follows on wrongly conducted physical exercise. It is here spontaneously occurring, however, and will often constitute pain."

The Byzantine Christian physician, Aetius, commenting upon this fragment of Theophrastus' thesis, *On Lassitude*, advised that treatment could generally only be
given successfully if it were applied at the very onset of
an attack. He recommended an initial purge, to be followed by inunction with hot or cold liniments, preferably
by two vigorous operators at the same time. If the onset
were accompanied with severe headache, or haemorrhage,
the patient must be bled in order to prevent the onset of
fever. He also mentioned the fatty tissues as being spe-
cially subject to pain of this type. An acute form with

local heat and fever, which he described, may perhaps have been cellulitis.

After the fall of the Roman Empire medicine became increasingly academic and withdrawn; Moslem and mediaeval physicians, wedded to their texts and their commentaries, seldom found it necessary to come into personal touch with their patients. In these circumstances a loose, indeterminate category of non-articular pains of this sort, although common, found no place or identifiable name in medical writings until the time of the European Renaissance.

Jerome Cardan referred in his commentaries on the aphorisms of Hippocrates to this forgotten group of maladies. He tells us nothing new about them, however, reiterating only the words of the Master. Following this lead of Cardan we find Jean Fernel, Henry II of France's great physician, resuscitating the conception and ascribing it in his *Pathologia* (1554) to "that superfluous humour which percolates under the skin deeply below the surface of the body outside the joints," and which the organism is for some reason unable to void, "thus causing many and great pains in many places." He thought that a similar pathology would cause visceral pain, so that he felt bound, as we now do, to regard "the skin and tissues which limit the confines of the body" as an organ in the physiological sense of the word.

We then come to the *Liber de Rhumatismo* of Guillaume de Baillou (1642), in which he described, in addition to the various categories of gout and arthritis, a class of pains which might or might not be associated with fever and joint swelling. To this category he attached for the first time the name "rheumatism." He mentioned that in addition to this there existed a large unclassifiable collection of "pains of a catarrhal nature analogous to arthritis," but localised more superficially, and suggested that "those tissues which constitute the coverings of the body may also, like the viscera, have their special functions, their health and their diseases." He postulated a failure of the skin in its function as an excretory organ and the accumulation of acid humours to cause these pains. He said of the rheumatism and of the non-articular pains that "they appear to be so nearly related that they are like two sisters"; but later reverted to the old terminology of Theophrastus referring to the latter group collectively as "idiopathic lassitude."

One of his disciples, Rondelet, was more fanciful in his belief—which is quoted by Delpeuch—that non-articular pains are caused by an overflow of the excess humour from the deep viscera, impinging violently upon the outer regions of the body, "fiercely, like the waves which surge out of a river bed when after a heavy rain it can no longer contain them, and the country far afield is suddenly deluged."

Felix Plater, the Swiss physician whose attractive diary of his student days in Montpellier was recently published in English translation, wrote a textbook, *Praxeos Medicae* (1603), in which he classified pain into many categories. One of these was "that which affects the soft tissues lying between the skin and the internal organs of the body," such as lumbago, torticollis, and pleurodynia. Friedrich Hoffmann (1660–1742), commenting later upon these views, wrote (1729): "Those illustrious French doctors defined as 'rheumatic' those pains which fleetingly affect the limbs, the muscles of the neck, the arm, the front and back of the thorax, shoulders, thighs and hands. Only those which localise in the joints do they call arthritic." He then proceeded to extend this concept by suggesting the inclusion of a number of other types of pain, including muscle spasm, scorbutic, venereal, dental, and other pains, which would not seem to us today to merit the adjective "rheumatic." In this way he started the modern habit of referring to any pain for which cause is not apparent as "a touch of rheumatism."

Thus the concept of a migration of body fluid into soft tissues of the body causing non-articular pain was finally established; but interest was not maintained, as further classification of the resulting pain syndromes seemed unprofitable.

Sydenham had also referred to pains of non-articular type in his *Treatise on the Gout* (1683). He classified them as "other kinds of scorbutical rheumatisms," a subterfuge to separate them aetiologically from gout and chronic arthritis without committing himself further. Of this group he said: "The pain seizes sometimes this part, sometimes that, but seldom occasions swelling; neither is it accompanied by a fever, nor is it fixt for long, but is more of a wandering nature and has irregular and disorderly symptoms; now it afflicts this or that member, by and by it seizes the inward parts and occasions sickness which goeth off again when the pain returns to the outward parts; and so afflicts the patient by turns and continues a long while." He mentioned the belief that such pains, particularly when they occurred in the spring, could be cured with "sweete wholesome butter," which perhaps reinforces his scorbutic attribution. A well-authenticated example of scorbutic rheumatism is to be found in the diary of the antarctic explorer Captain Scott, who mentions that many of his party began to suffer severely with rheumatism shortly before their death, which was almost certainly the result of scurvy.

Sydenham's pupil, Boerhaave, took the matter a little further when he said of rheumatism later that: "If fixing itself in the loins it deserves the name of lumbago; if in the thighbone it is called the sciatica or hip-gout. They are cured by the same methods or means, but not so easily."

Sciatica

References to sciatica will be found in the works of Hippocrates, whose sixteenth aphorism, for instance, states: "In persons afflicted with 'the hip-gout,' if the bone grows out round the socket of the joint the limb becomes wasted and maimed unless the part be cauterised." He continued: "If the pain be fixed in the leg and does not yield to medicines, burn it with flax." This advice was echoed nearly two thousand years later by the great surgeon, John Arbuthnot, who said: "In obstinate sciatical pains blistering and cauteries are the most effectual treatment." The Byzantine physician, Rufus of Ephe us, wrote a tract on this disorder, but the only original information which he contributed is that: "The Scythians using continual riding were generally molested with the sciatica," a matter which was further examined by Sir Thomas Browne in his *Vulgar Errors* in the seventeenth century.

In Tudor England Dr. Andrew Boorde referred to it as "ye sciaticke passion," and said that it was a variety of podagra settling round the hip joint and that "it passes in time!" Fernel had a deeper understanding which is thought to have been born of personal suffering. In his *Pathologia* (1554) he remarked: "Sciatica is one of the most violent of pains, and is not only situated in the joint but is also deeper in the upper part of the buttocks at that point where the lumbar and sacral nerves enter the thigh. It is an appalling pain, which does not confine itself to the leg, but extends down the thigh right into the foot—everywhere in fact where the sciatic nerve *in nervo lato* extends its branches." This was written two hundred years before Domenico Cotugno (1736–1822) published in Naples his little book *De Ischiade Nervosa Commentarius* (1764), for which he is generally given priority concerning implication of the nerve itself in this condition. Cotugno described two forms: the one in which the pain results from an inflammation in or around the hip joint; the other, the "ischias nervosa," or true sciatic neuritis in which pain is caused by swelling or irritation of the sheath of the nerve. The causes he stated to be cold, injury, or "the rheumatic virus." S. A. Tissot of Lausanne also tells us (1793) how he cured his own long-standing sciatica with a plaster of quicklime and honey blended together: "This did also raise a little vesication of the parts."

William Heberden, in his *Commentaries*, wrote on the treatment of sciatica and lumbago, which he believed to be manifestations of gout, as did most authorities until fifty years ago; and after discussing the relative virtues of cold and hot bathing, blistering, cupping, and purging, declared: "Opium, notwithstanding Sydenham's objections, has at least proved a safe and effective remedy for the purpose of mitigating the pain, and of procuring easy nights of sleep. . . . Time and warm bathing and flannel may contribute a little to the cure or relief." He reminds us of Shakespeare's malediction in *Timon of Athens:*

> Thou cold *Sciatica,*
> Cripple our Senators, that their limbs may halt
> As lamely as their manners.

His friend and patient, Dr. Samuel Johnson, was a sufferer, and gave it as his opinion that "The sciatic pain, Sir, is the most diabolic to which man may be subjected."

General James Wolfe suffered frequent bouts throughout his short life, and these had important repercussions if, as his biographer maintains, it was his desperate effort to live down this affliction that constituted the mainspring of his energies in creating Canada.

During the nineteenth century François Valleix (1807–1855) of Paris recorded (1841) his observation concerning the localised tender spots which occur in the course of the sciatic nerve, the "puncta dolorosa," which still bear his name; and E. C. Lasègue (1816–1883), who was also the first to describe the condition known as "anorexia nervosa," developed his well-known diagnostic leg-raising sign. Nothing further of note occurred until about 1911, when the French physician, Jean Sicard (1872–1929), Widal's favourite pupil, together with Henri Forestier of Aix, first established the spinal origin of both sciatica and lumbago, as did independently the Italian surgeon, Vittorio Putti (1880–1940). They failed to discern the importance of the intervertebral discs in these matters, however.

The intervertebral disc had been described by the anatomist, Vesalius, in the sixteenth century and its minute structure and embryology by H. Luschka of Berlin in 1858. Professor Schmörl of Dresden described in 1927 displacements of this structure which he had found in autopsy material, but the fact that it could be displaced by accident or disease during life and so cause sciatica and lumbago was discovered and developed independently by Middleton and Teacher in Glasgow and by Goldthwait in Boston. These observers described cases in which the disc had either herniated or slipped backwards, and so partially compressed the spinal cord in similar fashion to a tumour. It became possible soon afterwards to remove such prolapsed discs surgically, and the American surgeon, Barr, published successful results in fifty-three cases in 1937; whilst in 1945 a splendid report by Glenn Spurling of his many hundred cases seen during the war in Europe was published and put the subject onto a firm basis.

Non-Articular Rheumatism in the Services

Through the eighteenth century we find but little reference in academic works to non-articular rheumatism. In the *Observations on the Practice of the Westminster General Dispensary* (1777), Dr. John Miller reported that of the 2,553 patients admitted during its first two years there were many cases of rheumatism, and in 189 of these he noted that the joints were unaffected. But most hospital reports are silent on this subject. The armed forces, however, had to take a realistic view of a syndrome which, although difficult to classify, was wont to deplete their effective manpower for considerable periods. It is thus to such works as Sir John Pringle's *Diseases of the Army* (1752) that we must turn for information.

Pringle stated, as have medical historians in our time, that "rheumatism is one of the most frequent diseases of the Army, especially at the beginning of a campaign." In the first three weeks of 1704, he said, two hundred and fifty soldiers were admitted to hospital; of these seventy-one were suffering with pneumonia and pleurisy and seventy-six with "rheumatism."

Again, during the campaign of 1743 which culminated in the battle of Fontenoy, he reported that "sickness was moderate and we sent into hospital not above 1/43rd part of the army. When the number was 220 the distempers were classed and stood as follows: pleurises and peripneumonies 71, rheumatic pains with more or less of fevers,

57, rheumatic pains without fevers 25 . . . this with little variation was the state of the camp diseases." He pointed out that officers were not so subject to the rheumatic pains as the common man, being less exposed; and for a like reason the cavalry: "for the care of the horses gives the men an easy but constant employment, and their cloaks serve for bed clothes at night."

Dr. Donald Monro (1737–1802) of St. George's Hospital, who had accompanied the Duke of Marlborough upon his campaigns, later wrote *Observations on the Means of Preserving the Health of Soldiers* (1780), and observed that "in the Army, even in its milder forms, the chronic rheumatism is one of the most obstinate of diseases to be cured. . . . There were at all times men in our hospitals, labouring under rheumatic complaints; but we had few of the rheumatisms accompanied with swellings, pain and inflammation of the joints, which are so common in our hospitals about London."

He reports interestingly upon a number of cases which had resisted his treatment with repeated drastic purging and daily cold baths. In this course he was probably following the method which had been advocated by Dr. John Cheshire of Leicester, himself a sufferer, in his book *A Treatise upon the Rheumatism, as well Acute as Chronicall* (1735), who said that: "In slight and chronic rheumatic complaints which do not confine a patient to his bed, there is not a more expeditious and certain relief than plunging him into cold water, and thereafter to get him betwixt a pair of blankets." He particularly recommended this for sciatic pain: ". . . and by bathing him in the Sea." No doubt the use of such methods in the Army also exercised some deterrent effect upon potential malingerers.

In his book referred to above, Sir John Pringle mentioned that malingerers were then, as in more recent times, a feature of army medical life. He suggested that soldiers who reported sick on account of rheumatism, but who had little to show for it, should be bled to see whether or not a "buffy coat" appeared upon the blood's surface. "If the blood be not found sizy we may presume that the soldier either pretends indisposition, or that the pains are of another nature." This is, of course, a primitive way of performing the modern erythrocyte sedimentation-rate-test (ESR), and would not in fact prove infallible. This Pringle realised later in life when he wrote: "I have since seen patients with these same complaints, under no temptation to deceive, without alteration in their blood."

Donald Monro corroborated the view that "there is no disorder which soldiers are so apt to counterfeit as the rheumatic whenever the duty in the field is severe; but when there is no fever, or size in the blood, or other marks of distemper, and the man looks healthy, there is always reason to suspect imposture."

We also have the testimony of Dr. William Balfour of Edinburgh that non-articular rheumatism was equally common during the Peninsular War. He wrote (1816): "I have been informed by all the military gentlemen of my acquaintance that more men are invalided from rheumatism than from all other diseases combined. . . . In a retreat in particular, after the Army had toiled all day in the burning sun and laid themselves down at night upon the cold ground, many were unable in the mornings to make use of their arms."

If we look through contemporary army medical reports we can learn something of the size of the problem these undramatic but disabling aches and pains provided for the regimental medical officers. We can read, for instance, that in 1703 "several diseases were common among the men of the 29th Regiment in Chatham Barracks, and the West Indies, such as rheumatism . . . this was not attended with such severe symptoms as were seen in our Army in America." The returns for this regiment, which seem rather high, were given later in tabular form:

1780 Rheumatism 35—total sick 660.
1781 Rheumatism 28—total sick 464.
1782 Rheumatism 28—total sick 299.

The navy too had its rheumatic problem. Dr. Robert Robertson, surgeon in Admiral Geary's flagship, "Edgar," during the American War of Independence, records that from July 1779, to May 1782, the sick list comprised "Fevers 689, Wounded 91, Rheumatism 84," whilst James Lind's nosological list for his first two years as physician in charge of the Haslar Hospital at Plymouth shows: "Scurvy 1,146, Consumption 360, Rheumatism 350." On the North African Station in Lord Howe's flagship, "Juno," which was described as being exceptionally healthy (1776–1778), the list shows "Fevers 514, Dysentery 83, and Rheumatism 59." Sickness returns for the Crimean War showed that of 29,310 admissions to hospital 3,560 were for rheumatism, of whom eight died. In 1900 these figures were similar as *The Incidence of General Diseases in the Navy* informs us that the number of ratings invalided for this reason (2,932) was third only to influenza and venereal disease.

Nelson's surgeon, Sir William Beatty, tells us that the Admiral enjoyed excellent health in the weeks preceding the battle of Trafalgar, except for twinges of gout or rheumatism, which he overcame by a strict diet and renunciation of salt. Writing from the "Victory" in January 1805, Nelson himself mentioned that consumption and rheumatism were the only two serious complaints in his fleet at that time.

At a somewhat earlier period the question of flannel seems to have become a controversial issue. Admiral Sir William Dillon, writing of the action of "the Glorious 1st of June," mentions that his surgeon, James Malcolm, who lost his nerve after the battle and had to leave the service, was "an amiable man who was the cause of introducing flannel for the use of seamen to protect them against the effects of rheumatism." His Commander-in-Chief, Lord St. Vincent, approved this idea, and ordered (1794) that "in cold weather flannel shall be worn next the skin." He went on to "exhort most sincerely the Captains of the ships comprising the fleet under my command to inculcate this doctrine in the minds of your surgeons, who from caprice and perverse opposition to every wholesome regulation grossly neglect this important duty." The physician to the fleet, Dr. Thomas Trotter, no sooner heard this, however, than he sent a violent protest to the Admiral, saying that the men would perspire greatly in the course of their duties and being unable to wash or dry themselves "would have to steam themselves dry in their hammocks. . . . Clothe them as warm as you like," he added, "but give them linen or cotton next the skin." History does not record the outcome of this quarrel, although the two men never met again as Trotter retired soon after into civilian life.

Non-articular rheumatism remains a large problem today in civilian life. It was shown by a recent British survey that one in fifty men and women in industry are disabled annually for four to six weeks and that twenty-seven million working days are lost each year to industry as the result of it.

Prevention

Although Sydenham had believed that rheumatism is

an Act of God, which must be endured, Pringle was not
of this opinion and he made a number of very sensible
preventive suggestions to the Army Council. Amongst
these was the provision of an extra clothing issue for
soldiers on active service in winter, and a supply of under-
waistcoats for all ranks, with overcoats in addition for
sentries; also an issue of blankets for every tent. He advised that fuel be provided to dry their clothes; but their
bodies, he thought, should dry as the result of exercise.
All these matters were first put to trial in the campaign
of 1745 in the Highlands of Scotland, against "Bonnie
Prince Charlie," the Society of Friends providing the
necessary flannel. As the weather was very cold there was
little temptation for the men to sleep on the grass, which
Pringle thought was often a major cause of their rheumatic troubles.

In the civilian memoirs of the celebrated Reverend
Sydney Smith we find him writing, about 1820: "It is
lamentable to see how ignorant the rural poor are about
the common affairs of life." He accordingly followed this
up by writing a pamphlet giving practical advice on many
subjects, which he distributed amongst his parishioners.
One of the early paragraphs begins:

> Never sit in wet clothes! Off with them as soon as you
> can; no constitution can stand it. Look at Jackson who lives
> next door to the blacksmith: he was the strongest man in
> the parish. Twenty different times I warned him of his
> folly. He was very civil, but clearly seemed to think it all
> old women's nonsense. He is now, as you can see, bent
> double with rheumatism, and is scarcely able to crawl from
> pillar to post!

Causation

Apart from trauma and cold it was thought by some of
our predecessors, as by many authorities today, that non-

articular rheumatism could be caused purely by mental stress; in the modern United States "psychogenic rheumatism" is often used as a synonym. In the first great classification of disease, the *Nosologica Methodica* (1763) of Sauvages, chronic rheumatism was subdivided into fifteen further varieties, of which "rhumatismus hystericus" seems to refer to acute muscular rheumatism. A further precedent for this psychiatric view can be found in the works of Sydenham, who wrote: "Thus it harrasses the patient by turns, and prolongs itself to the duration of the most chronick of diseases . . . were it not for its resistance to hysteric remedies, it might pass for a sort of hysteria." However, Heberden, with gentle cynicism, disposed of all such hypotheses with his dictum that "Rheumatism is but a common name for many aches and pains which have as yet achieved no particular designation."

Towards the end of the eighteenth century Dr. William Falconer of Bath observed (1795) that "those who work in mines of coal or of any other minerals and others employed where moisture is much concerned, are particularly liable to this disease." He also recognised—ahead of his time—the influence of certain heavy industries and of bad housing and suggested that improvement in environmental conditions might reduce its incidence.

In 1802 Philippe Pinel, physician to the Salpêtrière Hospital in Paris, became interested in a series of his patients who were suffering with "rheumatic" muscular pains and some fever. Two of these died, and post-mortem examination revealed numerous small abscesses in the muscles (mysositis). It was soon realised, however, that this finding was not typical of most cases of non-articular rheumatism as he at first thought. Hermann Senator summed up the causes as follows (1877): "It is a painful disorder of the somatic tissues due either to chill or to causes which cannot yet be ascertained, and are therefore generally presumed to be atmospheric in their aetiology." There are in fact a number of different forms of non-articular rheumatism, and the cause of each is different and sometimes unknown.

Treatment

In mediaeval times St. Gregory was decreed as the patron of all rheumatic sufferers, and rings and medallions bearing his effigy, and blessed by some suitably holy man, were much used both for prophylactic and therapeutic purposes. So-called cramp rings were also worn for the relief of rheumatic pains—much as are copper bracelets today—and were said to have been devised by King Edward the Confessor who distributed them to those in need of such relief, "without money or petition." This practice was continued by subsequent monarchs, including Henry VIII. With the rise of science in the seventeenth century, iodine, sulphur, and other chemical lockets came into favour for a similar purpose. Like most irregular therapy all this perhaps constituted a triumph of hope over experience.

Orthodox medical treatment did not distinguish between articular and non-articular varieties of rheumatism until modern times. In the eighteenth century Cullen and some others advocated, for those who remained mobile, that rare adventure: a hot bath, "with the plentiful application of the flesh-brush to the afflicted area." The cold-water cure of Dr. Cheshire has already been mentioned, and as a possible alternative in humble circles, "flogging with weeds of stinging nettle." During the eighteenth and nineteenth centuries, and even before, affluent patients would flock to the "Spaws" for thermal-water or mud treatment. George III's banker, "honest Tom Coutts," wrote that: "At Christmas time, in spite of the weather, I always go to Buckstone to be boiled for the rheumatism," and readers of Smollett's novel *Humphrey Clinker,* will recall his revealing descriptions of the fashionable treatment at Bath. It was for the purpose of taking patients from their lodgings to the medicinal baths that the "Bath chair" was designed. Smollett mentions that these special sedan chairs "stand soaking all day and night in the streets until they have become so many boxes of wet leather for the greater benefit of the gouty and the rheumatic."

When Dr. James Graham's licentious "Temple of Health" (in which Nelson's love, Emma Hamilton, as a girl is said to have made her debut) became bankrupt in 1782, Graham tried to restore its fortunes by introducing mud baths—both single and double—"for the treatment of the slighter pains of rheumatism and gout." He used to demonstrate their pleasurable harmlessness by spending many hours in them himself and even giving public lectures from this curious vantage point. He may have obtained his idea from a very successful charlatan named Alessandro Domenichetti, who claimed to be of noble Venetian birth and who ran a vapour-bath establishment in Chelsea. Domenichetti pretended by "analysis" to recognise certain deficiencies in the blood of sufferers which he could replace by adding the necessary substance to the steam. This, he said, would carry it into the innermost recesses of the body. He numbered the Royal Family and most of the celebrities of his time amongst his patients and initiated a cult which exists to this day.

Spa treatment has always consisted in "taking the waters" as well as external application, and in time a visit in person was considered by some to be an unnecessary fatigue for the rheumatic sufferer. Consequently bottles of reputed spa water were sent by carriers all over the country. Dr. Johnson of Malvern, for instance, advertised the advantages of his local bottled water—in which he had a share-holding—over the prescriptions of ordinary doctors, "who dropped drugs of which they knew little into stomachs of which they knew less"; and advocated a graduated course of hydrotherapeutic home treatment. The bottled "Natural medicated spring-water cure for home use" also became "big business" in the United States throughout the last century.

Rational do-it-yourself therapy seems to have found its apogee in the person of the Reverend Sydney Smith, the celebrated political writer and wit, and his "rheumatic Armour." This he kept in a large bag in his study and would demonstrate to all his callers. One of these wrote:

> You must fancy him in a fit of his rheumatism; his legs in two narrow buckets which he calls his Jack boots; round the throat a hollow tin collar: over each shoulder a large tin thing like a leg of mutton; on his head a hollow tin helmet and a breastplate and stomacher, all filled with hot water. He says that the stomach-tin is the greatest comfort in life.

Massage was introduced for the treatment of non-articular rheumatism towards the middle of the century, largely as the result of the Berlin surgeon Robert Froriep's conception of its cause being the development of "fibroid patches, or indurations, in the muscles or in the fibrous tissues overlying them." He thought that in favourably early cases these could be dispersed by deep friction. His ideas were published in 1843, *De Rheumatische Schwielen.*

Then came the phase in which an hidden focus of in-

fection was postulated and removed. One verse of a somewhat cynical poem written by an American sufferer in
1920 seems adequately to summarise the contemporary
situation:

> Sometimes we yank the tonsils, and sometimes we yank the
> teeth,
> (In hope that there are foci of infection there beneath).
> Sometimes we wash the sinus; and sometimes that helps it
> too;
> But sometimes we merely wonder what the devil we can do.

Today, treatment of non-articular rheumatism is
largely based upon general measures and the intelligent
use of aspirin and its variants. In addition to this a
proper use of diet and exercise, and the help of modern
forms of physiotherapy, will generally serve to prevent
the victim of these disorders from having to embark
upon any of the wilder forms of orthodox or unorthodox
quackery which offered little but hope to his forefathers.
The present therapeutic situation seems an improvement
upon Osler's favourite regime for "fibrositis" which as
he recorded, only fifty years ago, was "Hope and Nux
Vomica in moderate dosage."

We may perhaps end our book with a quotation from
a leading article which appeared in the *Times* of London
some years ago, which the present writer hopes may help
to justify the historical labours here recorded: "It is always sad to read of the belittlement of our great ancestors," it declared, "who, surrounded by so many obstacles,
trod their laborious path and followed it to its bright
consummation in contemporary medical science. . . .
History in Greek means 'investigation,' not 'chronicle,'
and modern medical problems can only be understood
in the light of their historical origin and development."

To do just this has been the object of this book. The history of medicine, far from being, as some think, a chronicle of the follies and errors of our crude ancestors, is the study and record of the progressive development of what has been thought to be the noblest conquest of the human mind.

A Select Bibliography

Sufficient identification is given in the text of most of the works quoted there. Many other books and articles have also been consulted, of which the following list is representative.

Alexander of Tralles. *Oeuvres Médicales*. Paris: Geuthner, 1933–1937. 4 vols.

Aretaeus the Cappadocian. *The Extant Works*. Edited and translated by Francis Adams. London: The Sydenham Society, 1856.

Aschoff, Karl Albert Ludwig. "Zur Myocarditisfrage," *Verhandlungen der Deutschen Pathologischen Gesellschaft*, 1904, 8: 46–53.

Baillou, Guillaume de. *Liber de Rhumatismo*. Paris: J. Quesnel, 1642. Translated into English by C. C. Barnard, *British Journal of Rheumatism*, 1940, 2: 141–162.

Balfour, William. *Observations, with Cases Illustrative of a New, Simple, and Expeditious Mode of Curing Gout*. Edinburgh: J. & C. Muirhead, 1816.

Barlow, Sir Thomas, and Francis Warner. "On Subcutaneous Nodules Connected with the Fibrous Structures Occurring in Children the Subjects of Rheumatism and Chorea," *Transactions of the International Medical Congress, 7 session, held in London, 2–9 August 1881*. London: 1881, vol. 4 p. 46 ff.

Bechterev, Vladimir M. "Steifigkeit der Wirbelsäule und ihre Verkrümmung als besondere Erkrankungsform," *Neurologisches Centralblatt*, 1893, 12: 426–434.

Bett, Walter Reginald. *The History and Conquest of Common Diseases*. Norman, Oklahoma: University of Oklahoma Press, 1954.

Bick, Edgar Milton. *Source Book of Orthopaedics*. Baltimore: Williams & Wilkins, 1948.

Blackmore, Sir Richard. *Discoures on the Gout, Rheumatism, and the King's-Evil*. London: 1726.

Boerhaave, Hermann. *Dr. Boerhaave's Academical Lectures on the Theory of Physic*. London: 1757–1763. 6 vols.

Boorde, Andrew. *The Breviary of Healthe.* London: Thomas East, 1575.

Bouchard, Charles-Jacques. *Traité de Pathologie Générale.* Paris: 1895.

Boyle, Hon. Robert. *The Works.* London: 1772. 6 vols.

Bridges, Robert. "A Severe Case of Rheumatic Fever Treated Successfully by Splints," *Saint Bartholomew's Hospital Reports,* 1876, 12: 175–181.

Bywaters, E. G. L. "Gout in the Time and Person of George IV," *Annals of the Rheumatic Diseases,* 1962, 21: 325–338.

Caelius Aurelianus. *On Acute Diseases, and on Chronic Diseases.* Edited and translated by I. E. Drabkin. Chicago: University of Chicago Press, 1950.

Celsus. *On Medicine.* Translated by James Grieve. London: 1755.

Chauffard, Anatole, and Félix Ramond. "Des Adénopathies dans le Rhumatisme Chronique Infectieux," *Revue de Médecine,* 1896, 16: 345–359.

Cheshire, John. *A Treatise upon the Rheumatism, as well Acute as Chronical.* London: J. Rivington, 1735.

Connor, Bernard. "An Extract of a Letter from Bernard Connor, M.D., to Sir Charles Walgrave, Published in French at Paris: Giving an Account of an Extraordinary Humane Skeleton, Whose Vertebrae of the Back, the Ribs, and Several Bones down to the Os Sacrum, Were All Firmly United into One Solid Bone, without Joynting or Cartilage," *Philosophical Transactions of the Royal Society,* 1695, 19: 21–27.

Copeman, W. S. C. *Doctors and Disease in Tudor Times.* London: Dawson's of Pall Mall, 1961.

———. *Textbook of the Rheumatic Diseases.* Edinburgh: Livingstone, 1964. (Sections on history and classification.)

Costa, Antonio, and Giorgio Weber, "Le Alterazioni Morbose del Sistema Scheletrico in Cosimo dei Medici il Vecchio, in Piero il Gottoso, in Lorenzo il Magnifico, in Giuliano Duca di Nemours," *Archivio "De Vecchi,"* 1955, 23: 1–69.

Dale, Philip Marshall. *Medical Biographies: The Ailments*

of *Thirty-three Famous Persons*. Norman, Oklahoma: University of Oklahoma Press, 1952.

Delpeuch, Armand. *La Goutte et le Rhumatisme*. Paris: G. Carré & C. Naud, 1900.

Donne, William Bodham. *Old Roads and New Roads*. London: 1852.

Duckworth, Sir Dyce. *A Treatise on Gout*. London: 1889.

Dumoulin, M. *Nouveau Traité du Rhumatisme et des Vapeurs*. Paris: L. d'Houry, 1710.

Ellis, H. Havelock. *Morals, Manners and Men*. London: Thinkers Library, 1939.

Fagge, C. Hilton. "A Case of Simple Synostosis of the Ribs to the Vertebrae, and of the Arches and Articular Processes of the Vertebrae Themselves, and also of One Hip-Joint," *Transactions of the Pathological Society of London*, 1877, 28: 201–208.

Falconer, William. *An Account of the Bath Waters in Rheumatic Cases*. Bath: 1795.

Forestier, Jacques. "Le Traitement des Polyarthrites Chroniques par les Sels d'Or. Résultats Cliniques et Contrôles Hématologiques," *Bulletins et Mémoires des Hôpitaux de Paris*, 1930, 46 (sér. 4): 273–280.

Frazer, Sir James. *The Golden Bough*. Part VI (The Scapegoat). London: 1913.

Galen. *The Writings of Hippocrates and Galen Epitomised by J. R. Cox*. Philadelphia: 1846.

Gerard, John. *The Herball or, Generall Historie of Plantes*. London: 1597. Enlarged and Amended by Thomas Johnson, 1633.

Glover, J. A. "The Incidence of Rheumatic Diseases," *Ministry of Health Reports on Public Health and Medical Subjects*. no. 23. London, 1924, p. 97 ff.

Goldthwait, Joel Ernest. "The Differential Diagnosis and Treatment of the So-called Rheumatoid Disease," *Boston Medical and Surgical Journal*, 1904, 151: 529–534.

Graham, Wallace, and K. M. Graham. "Our Gouty Past," *Canadian Medical Association Journal*, 1955, 73: 485–493.

Haig, Alexander. *Uric Acid as a Factor in the Causation of Disease.* London: 1892.

Hartley, Sir Harold, ed. *The Royal Society, Its Origins and Founders.* London: The Royal Society, 1950. (Article: Jonathan Goddard.)

Hench, Philip S., *et al. Rheumatism Reviews, 1935–1941 . . . Published Originally in the Annals of Internal Medicine, Volumes 8–15.* Amsterdam: Excerpta Medica Foundation, 1961.

Hippocrates. *The Genuine Works.* Translated by Francis Adams. London: The Sydenham Society, 1849. 2 vols.

Houdé, A. "De la Colchicine Cristallisée," *Comptes Rendus Hebdomadaires des Séances et Mémoires de la Société de Biologie,* 1884, 1 (sér. 8): 218–220.

Jameson, Eric. *The Natural History of Quackery.* London: 1961.

Klemperer, Paul, Abou D. Pollack, and George Baehr. "Diffuse Collagen Disease," *Journal of the American Medical Association,* 1942, 119 (pt. 1): 331–332.

Klinge, Friedrich. *Der Rheumatismus; pathologisch-anatomische und experimentell-pathologische Tatsachen und ihre Auswertung für ärztliche Rheumaproblem.* Munich: J. F. Bergmann, 1933.

Latham, John. *On Rheumatism and Gout.* London: T. N. Longman, 1796.

Léri, André. "La Spondylose Rhizomélique," *Revue de Médicine,* 1899, 19: 597–624.

Lloyd, Christopher, and J. L. S. Coulter. *Medicine and the Royal Navy.* Vol. III. Edinburgh: Livingstone, 1961.

Lucian of Samosata. *The Plays with an English Translation by A. M. Harmon.* London: W. Heinemann, 1913 ff. 8 vols.

Lyons, Philip M. "Remarkable Case of Rapid Ossification of the Fibro-cartilaginous Tissues, or Pure General Anchylosis," *Lancet,* 1831–1832, Vol. I, pp. 27–29.

MacLagan, Thomas John. *Rheumatism: Its Nature, Its Pathology, and Its Successful Treatment.* London: Pickering, 1881.

Marie, Pierre. "Sur la Spondylose Rhizomélique," *Revue de Médicine,* 1898, 18: 285–315.

Mettler, Cecilia Charlotte. *History of Medicine.* Philadelphia: Blakiston, 1947.

Meynet, P. "Rhumatisme Articulaire Subaigu," *Lyon Médicale,* 1875, 19: 495–499.

Mitchell, J. K. "On a New Practice in Acute and Chronic Rheumatism," *The American Journal of the Medical Sciences,* 1831, No. XV, pp. 55–64.

Morel-Fatio, A., ed. *Mémoires de Charles-Quint.* Paris: 1913.

Morley, Henry. *Life of Jerome Cardan.* London: 1854. 2 vols.

Nichols, E. H., and F. L. Richardson. "Arthritis Deformans," *The Journal of Medical Research,* 1909, 21: 149 ff.

O'Connell, D. "Ankylosing Spondylitis. The Literature up to the Close of the Nineteenth Century," *Annals of the Rheumatic Diseases,* 1956, 15: 119–123.

Pagel, Walter. *Paracelsus. An Introduction to Philosophical Medicine in the Era of the Renaissance.* Basel: Karger, 1958.

Parkinson, Sir John. *Rheumatic Fever and Heart Disease. The Harveian Oration, 1945.* London: 1945.

Paul of Aegina. *The Seven Books.* Translated by Francis Adams. London: The Sydenham Society, 1844. 3 vols.

Pellétier, Pierre Joseph, and Joseph-Bienaimé Caventou. "Examen Chimique de Plusieurs Végétaux de la Famille des Colchicées et du Principe Actif qu'ils Renferment," *Annales de Chimie et de Physique,* 1820, 14: 69–83.

Pinel, Philippe. *La Médecine Clinique.* Paris: 1802.

Poncet, Antonin, and René Leriche. *Le Rhumatisme Tuberculeux.* Paris: 1909.

Poynton, Frederic John, and Alexander Paine. *Researches on Rheumatism.* London: J. & A. Churchill, 1913.

———, and Bernard Edward Schlesinger. *Recent Advances in the Study of Rheumatism.* London: J. & A. Churchill, 1937.

Reiter, Hans. "Ueber eine bisher unerkannte Spirochäten infektion (Spirochaetosis arthritica)," *Deutsche Medizinische Wochenschrift,* 1916, 42: 1535–1536.

Rufus of Ephesus. *Oeuvres.* Trad. par Charles Daremberg

et Charles Émile Ruelle. Paris: Imprimerie Nationale, 1879.

Scheele, Karl Wilhelm. *Chemical Essays.* Translated by T. Beddoes. London: Murray, 1786.

Smith, Sir Grafton Elliot. *The Archaeological Survey of Nubia. Report of 1907–1908.* Vol. II. Cairo: National Printing Department, 1910.

Spender, John Kent. *The Early Symptoms and the Early Treatment of Osteo-Arthritis (Commonly Called Rheumatoid Arthritis).* London: H. K. Lewis, 1889.

Still, Sir George Frederick. "On a Form of Chronic Joint Disease in Children," *Medico-Chirurgical Transactions,* 1896–1897, 80: 47–59.

Stone, Rev. Edmund. "An Account of the Success of the Bark of the Willow in the Cure of Agues," *Philosophical Transactions of the Royal Society,* 1763, 53: 195–200.

Strangeways, T. S. P., and J. B. Burt. "A Study of Skiagrams from the Hands of 100 Cases of So-called Rheumatoid Arthritis and Chronic Gout," *Reports of the Committee for the Study of Special Diseases.* Edinburgh, 1905, Vol. I, pp. 145–164.

Strümpell, Adolf. "Bermerkungen über die chronische ankylosirende Entzündung der Wirbelsäule und der Hüftgelenke," *Deutsche Zeitschrift für Nervenheilkunde,* 1897, 11: 338–342.

Talbott, John H. "The Treatment of Gout," *Bulletin of the New York Academy of Medicine,* 1942, 18 (ser. 2): 318–328.

Temple, Sir William. *An Essay on the Cure of the Gout.* London: 1681.

Turberville, Arthur Stanley, ed. *Johnson's England.* Oxford: Clarendon Press, 1933. 2 vols.

Ure, Alexander. "Researches on Gout," *London Medical Gazette,* 1844–1845, 35: 188–195.

Van Swieten, Gerard. *The Commentaries upon the Aphorisms of Dr. Herman Boerhaave.* London: 1759–1765. 14 vols.

Walpole, Hon. Horace. *Letters.* Edited by Lord Macauley. London: 1833.

Weintraud, W. "Die Behandlung der Gicht mit Phenylchi-
nolincarbonsäure (Atophan) nebst Bermerkungen über
die diätetische Therapie der Krankheit," *Die Therapie
der Gegenwart*, 1911, 13 (New ser.) : 97–105.

West, Samuel. "Analysis of Forty Cases of Rheumatic Fever,"
Saint Bartholomew's Hospital Reports, (1878), 14: 221–
233.

Willcox, Sir W. H. "Focal Sepsis," *Reports on Chronic
Rheumatic Diseases*. London, H. K. Lewis, 1935, Vol. I,
p. 72 ff.

Wollaston, William Hyde. "On Gouty and Urinary Concretions," *Philosophical Transactions of the Royal Society*,
1787, 77: 386 ff.

Wootton, A. C. *Chronicles of Pharmacy*. London: Mac-
millan, 1910. 2 vols.

Young, George Frederick. *The Medici*. New York: The
Modern Library, 1930.

Index

Lightning Source UK Ltd.
Milton Keynes UK
UKHW010656051221
395058UK00003B/263